T0368404

The Natural Menopause Handbook

THE NATURAL MENOPAUSE HANDBOOK

REVISED

Herbs, Nutrition & Other Natural Therapies

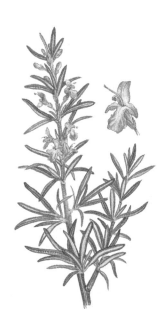

AMANDA McQUADE CRAWFORD, RH (AHG), MNIMH

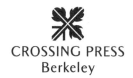

CROSSING PRESS
Berkeley

This book is dedicated to my daughter, Nora Serena, whom conventional medicine predicted I could never have. May she know the strength of women and the healing power of nature so that all her life changes are graceful. To all women and men who heal, and to the plants that steward animal, human, and planetary health, I am grateful and in your debt.

Copyright © 2009 by Amanda McQuade Crawford

All rights reserved.
Published in the United States by Crossing Press, an imprint of the Crown Publishing Group, a division of Random House, Inc., New York.
www.crownpublishing.com
www.tenspeed.com

Crossing Press and the Crossing Press colophon are registered trademarks of Random House, Inc.

Library of Congress Cataloging-in-Publication Data
Crawford, Amanda McQuade.
  The natural menopause handbook : herbs, nutrition & other natural therapies / Amanda McQuade Crawford. —1st ed.
    p. cm.
  Rev. ed. of: Herbal menopause book. c1996.
  Includes bibliographical references and index.
  Summary: "Focuses on herbs, nutrition, and other natural approaches to offer a holistic plan for wellness during menopause"—Provided by publisher.
  1. Menopause—Alternative treatment. 2. Herbs—Therapeutic use. 3. Naturopathy. I. Crawford, Amanda McQuade. Herbal menopause book. II. Title.

RG186.C75 2009
618.1'75061—dc22

2009015835

ISBN 978-1-58091-196-2

Cover design by Chloe Rawlins
Text design by Lynn Bell, Monroe Street Studios

First Revised Edition

146028962

Contents

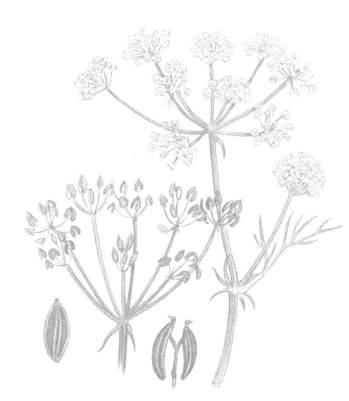

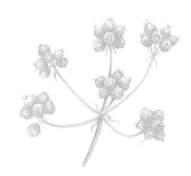

Foreword

*W*omen have always attended their mothers, sisters, and daughters through all the major transitions of life: birth, menarche, and menopause. Throughout history, much of this care was given outside the conventional medicine of the times and included a wide range of treatments such as herbs, foods, and hydrotherapy. This system of care (often passed from mother to daughter) declined as modern biomedicine grew in strength, giving us the miracles of safe childbirth, painless surgery, and effective drugs. Since the upsurge of the complementary and alternative medicine movement in the last half of the twentieth century, many women are once again asking to incorporate these gentle, natural therapies into their care. Despite the increasing numbers of women entering the health professions (and the army of nurses who have always been there), the biomedical system has been slow to incorporate these practices for a variety of reasons.

Happily, in this book, Amanda McQuade Crawford has bridged the biomedical and herbal traditions to give menopausal women sound advice that anchors the use of diet and herbal therapies in the context of modern biomedicine. This is the second edition of a book that has been a favorite of many women for more than ten years—and it's still timely now. Women need high-quality information placed in the correct context to make smart choices about their self-care as well as their health care. They need to know what lifestyle choices support their health and reduce risk. They need to know what tools they have to manage symptoms in effective, non-toxic ways. These needs are especially acute as women transition through menopause—a largely unappreciated change in Western culture.

For all these reasons and more, it gives me great pleasure to recommend Amanda McQuade Crawford's second edition to you. I hope that you find wisdom, health, and a new outlook on yourself. I also hope that you will bring this book with you when you see your biomedical practitioner and continue the critical dialogue that patients have brought to their care—patients should have the most effective, least toxic therapy possible. This book empowers women to discover such therapies in the pursuit of good health.

Mary L. Hardy, MD
May 2009

Acknowledgments

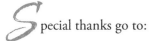pecial thanks go to:

- ❀ Mark McQuade Crawford, for many years of loving devotion and late-night fixes on my writing.

- ❀ My mother, Iris Jeanne McQuade, for first inspiring me to trust women's wisdom and the common sense in Nature.

- ❀ The several hundred women who placed their health in my care over twenty years of practicing the art of herbal medicine. It has been a privilege to have shared every one of your journeys. Each of you is my teacher.

- ❀ Bevin Clare and my teachers, mentors, and herbal friends and colleagues, for enriching my understanding of clinical practice in our complex, unpredictable culture.

- ❀ Sara Golski, my gifted, patient editor, for showing me uncommon courtesy as I revised this book while making a complete hash of deadlines.

- ❀ Kristi Hein, for her welcome balance of sensitive copyediting, precision, and encouragement.

- ❀ Aviva Jill Romm, MD, and Mary Hardy, MD, for their critical medical revisions of my material and for the uplifting friendships between our families. Our sisterhood nourishes my soul and you both make me laugh. Thank you.

- ❀ Joan Borysenko, PhD, for her life's work bringing rigorous science and spiritual reality into focus for the rest of us. Even before our first meeting years ago, your writing opened my eyes to potentials for integration, as well as the beauty of clear thinking while feeling bliss.

- ❀ The researchers—both known personally and those unknown but carefully studied by me—plus the clinicians, writers, and philosophers whose achievements inform my evolving practice.

Any errors are entirely mine. I also acknowledge that soon enough after this book is in print, statements in this book will be overturned by new truths as our collective pool of knowledge about women's health deepens. Still, I know the simplest pathways to wholeness when choosing food and herbs as medicine do not change. We just adapt to constant change within the flow of a vital force no words fully describe. For my communion with that fount of healing from the plants and from life itself, I acknowledge my debt and gratitude.

Amanda McQuade Crawford, RH (AHG), MNIMH
Los Angeles, California
2009

Introduction

Though many excellent books on menopause give herbal recommendations, no one book covers all the questions and concerns of the millions of women who are embarking on, experiencing, or moving past this major life transition. *The Natural Menopause Handbook* focuses on herbs, nutrition, and other natural approaches for perimenopause—the time leading up to and including the Change—and the postmenopausal years.

Why a new edition, and why now? The main reason is that women's health around the world is not static; hence, it is not the same as it was thirteen years ago when I first wrote *The Herbal Menopause Book*. Then, I wrote that hormone replacement therapy (HRT) was dangerous and often unnecessary. Now, that is old news. But even natural therapies for menopause that have been used for years have evolved dramatically. Conventional approaches and natural medicine are merging into strategies for "wellness." If it works and is safe, why call it "alternative" or "complementary"? If it causes more problems than it solves, why call it "medicine"?

Unless illness causes or accompanies menopause, the conventional medical view is that menopause may not require treatment. Yet prescriptions are still refilled for hormone therapy (also known as hormone replacement therapy). The reason given today is for relief of debilitating symptoms. Another reason women take these drugs that affect hormones is to prevent osteoporosis. Yet according to the National Women's Health Network (www.nwhn.org), "Women with greater economic resources and with health insurance that will pay for screening tests and drug prescriptions are being overscreened, overdiagnosed, and overtreated for osteoporosis." Women who do need screening and treatment are less likely to be identified and treated.

Globally, menopausal health screening varies by region and socioeconomic status. Though breast cancer rates in Africa and Asia are one-tenth of the rates in Europe and North America, worldwide rates are all rising. The hypothesis is that we are varyingly exposed to pollution, chemical landfills, nuclear power plants, and availability of HRT. There are also big differences among women around the globe and breast cancer risk. Two factors are the ways we eat and lifetime estrogen exposure. Excess estrogen is a risk for breast cancer. Differences in childbearing patterns play a role in lower overall estrogen exposure. In some societies, a younger age at first birth and more pregnancies is the norm, lowering a woman's lifetime estrogen exposure. Longer breastfeeding is a positive protective factor.

Most peri- or postmenopausal women are not taking hormones now, and of those who do start prescription HRT, over half stop within two years because of dissatisfaction and side effects.

In a follow-up to the 1990 United States Nurses' Study, a 40 percent increase in breast cancer was found among women between fifty and sixty-four years old who had been on HRT for five years or longer, and a 70 percent increase in women between sixty-five and sixty-nine. Before the more recent National Institutes of Health study was halted in 2002, only a few studies in the United States had shown that hormone replacement therapy increases breast cancer, in comparison with several studies conducted in European countries that showed a 1 to 30 percent increase in risk of breast cancer.

Still, you'd think enough had been written already on the subject. As of this writing, I found 29,586 results for menopause books on Amazon.com. These range from the cartoonish—*For Dumb Women, Tell Me What to Do, Am I Crazy?*, to the panicked and desperate—*Survive the Catastrophe, What You* Have *to Know, Info You Can't Live Without*, right through to the warm and thoughtful—*Pleasures of, Journaling through, Poetry About, Wisdom and Myth*. The list of titles goes on: no-nonsense menopause diets, ayurveda for midlife women, the macrobiotic solution to menopause, the ultimate anti-aging plan; overnight cures with bioidentical hormones, homeopathy, meditation, and exercise. There are those that are entire, complete, encyclopedic, the only book worth reading. All have an audience, which should relieve us of our concern about determining the right or wrong way to approach our own health questions at midlife and later. But still, the choices for women can seem a baffling mix of the good, the bad, and the sensational.

With this book, I hope to increase women's knowledge about the choices they have in natural therapies for menopausal conditions. Do we need better knowledge? Yes. Nearly three hundred women between forty to sixty years old were polled in a 2004 online survey. Among the findings:

❀ Almost three-quarters of the women surveyed said their doctors were their most trusted source of recommendations about menopause and alternative treatment.

❀ Almost one-half (45 percent) said that information provided by their doctors was conflicting and confusing.

❀ Thirty-seven percent reported the use of hormone therapy to treat menopause symptoms.

❀ Sixty percent of women on HRT discontinued it before treatment was complete.

❀ Seventy-four percent of women who discontinued HRT were not on any other kind of treatment.

❀ Use of alternative therapies, especially soy, was almost as prevalent as HRT.

❀ Reasons given for choosing an herbal product were:

  • Concern about hormone therapy safety (55 percent)

  • Desire to use a "natural" product (45 percent)

❋ Thirty-one percent reported using herbal remedies, including *Ginkgo biloba, Panax ginseng, Hypericum perforatum* (St. John's wort), and *Actaea racemosa* (black cohosh), formerly known as *Cimicifuga racemosa.*

The latest research (and media coverage!) focused on these and other natural ways to achieve hormonal balance is all relatively recent, and thus overwhelming to a woman who needs facts, not another sales pitch. Who can sort out the ever-changing controversies without getting a PhD or handing over one's health on trust? Neither extreme is required. Natural menopause *can* be simple when women have information. Which foods calm hot flashes? Are herbs for mood changes safe? This book is for women following conventional therapies who may seek an expanded view of their health-care options. It is also for women already well versed in the simplicity and efficacy of natural medicine. For all women and their health-care providers who are interested in using herbs during menopause but are unsure about how to go about it, this book provides new answers to old questions, and some age-old answers to new questions: What can herbal therapy do for menopausal women? Can herbs replace conventional Western medical therapy? If you need hormones, can prescription drugs and herbs be used together? These are among the questions women most commonly ask when they first consider trying natural remedies. The answers are all encouraging.

Natural medicine—especially herbal therapy—in contrast to conventional hormone replacement therapy, offers safer self-care options for common symptoms, along with the added confidence a woman feels from being in control of making her own health. In a very real way, herbs offer a woman the support of all nature. This support was tried and found to be valuable to many women before her, down through the ages, during their natural time of Change. Herbs, wise nutrition choices, and other therapies that have recently been termed "holistic" have in fact been practiced by women around the world since the Stone Age. We do not yet have documented studies of all our best healing plants and foods, but we have thousands of woman-years of use from which to learn. No toxic herbs are included in this book; some of the stronger herbs are quite safe for women to use at home as recommended in the specific formulas.

The use of either equine hormones (from horses) or synthetic hormones in conventional medical practice is based on the view that menopause is a deficiency of estrogen, among other hormones. This in turn is believed by some to be caused by a failure of the ovaries. Herbal medicine does not follow this biomedical approach. The failure of the drug approach to menopausal health points to the flaw in this assumption. In fact, when the ovaries decrease circulating levels of estrogen at this time of life, it is part of our bodies' design for self-preservation. Foods and herbs can work in concert with allopathic medicine. Often, natural approaches replace the need for drugs entirely. The strongest argument in favor of natural medicine is that, in contrast with conventional medicine, menopause is treated not as a disease but as a natural stage in the evolution of every woman's life—to be celebrated, not medicated.

This book devotes a chapter to each of four main areas of interest:

❀ Perimenopause

❀ Menopause

❀ The use of hormones

❀ Postmenopausal wellness

Each chapter includes discussions of conditions and their causes followed by natural health care: herbs, nutrition, and other helpful information for mind-body health.

Following these chapters are five brief sections of additional information and support. Appendix A provides guidelines for preparing herbs: how to brew a perfect pot of therapeutic herb tea, and how to make extracts, herbal oils, and all the herbal preparations described in this book. For the adventurous woman or one who already uses herbs, Appendix B explains how to make your own herbal menopause formula, just in case those in this book don't suit all your needs. Appendix C suggests herbs for your home medicine chest, and Appendix D shows images of many of the herbs used in this book. The Resources section lists herb suppliers, organizations, educational sources, and publications. The Bibliography includes publications I relied on in writing this book, as well as others that may be of further interest to you.

HOW TO USE THIS BOOK

Each explanation of a symptom, imbalance, or health challenge presented in this book is followed by an "Herbal Medicine" section that in most cases provides two formulas. These are usually very similar to each other. One is in the form of a concentrated extract (called a tincture) taken in small doses; this is often more convenient than brewing a pot of tea. The other uses the same or almost the same herbs, only as a tea (for those women seeking a low-cost and alcohol-free option). Some women mix and match herb teas that taste good with herb tinctures that work fast. Since tinctures are more concentrated than tea, tinctures work faster and we can take less of the herbs that don't taste good. These sections list the actions produced by each herb on the lines across from that specific herb.

If, for example, you need help with debilitating hot flashes or brutal mood swings, take the concentrated formula from this book to your nearest herb shop and buy the extracts off the shelf. The tea is often as effective and affordable over time, though it may not work fast enough for the headache or hot flash requiring immediate attention. Milder because it is extracted in hot water instead of alcohol, each gentle dose of herb tea adds up, over time, to longer-lasting health. Also, the extra water that tea provides gives your body more hydration. This means more freedom to take up what the body needs and excrete what it doesn't. Water-soluble herbal constituents are the mildest way to care for yourself. If you are sensitive to medications, you may prefer to start with teas. The tea recipes have been simplified and changed since the first edition to reflect new conditions in the global herb trade. The ethics of sustainability, environmental protection, and fair pricing matter as much as or more than new research.

As your symptoms come and go, you can, if you like, use either tea or concentrate (tincture). If needed, you may take both tea and concentrate at the same time; there is no risk of overdose if you follow the guidelines given in this book.

Note: Whether you have one menopausal symptom or twenty, choose the herbal formula that focuses on your worst symptom first. After years of clinical herbal practice helping women through the Change, I have found that, as a general rule, one formula addressing your worst symptom first will extend to relieve accompanying imbalances. The very word *Change* became a euphemism for menopause when women didn't feel comfortable talking about such things. Whether your family still treats sexual topics as taboo or you embrace the idea of transformation, keeping your herb formula simple is the key to this book.

Following the "Herbal Medicine" section for each health challenge, you'll find a "Nutrition" section that offers suggestions for whole foods that provide vitamins and minerals to address each particular health imbalance. If the challenge is one that's known to respond well to natural supplements, the appropriate supplements are listed, with doses as well. This is the most conservative aspect of the holistic treatment plan presented in this book because, in my opinion, less is often more when it comes to taking manufactured products; this is true even with even natural medicine. I encourage you to eat well and buy fewer products. There are other books encouraging more dependence on megadoses of super-nutrients, but I prefer to emphasize whole foods and can include only what my experience leads me to recommend. If readers are surprised by my omission of the latest popular cures, I beg your pardon. I view supplements as just that—*supplemental* to wise nutrition choices and safely monitored botanical balancing.

The "In Addition" section for each health issue provides other helpful natural therapies. Guided imagery and visualization have helped many women in my practice, and in these sections throughout the book I have included several to try. Also included are recipes for therapeutic external creams, salves, and herbal oils; specific exercises; and ideas for making positive changes in your daily life.

Although the recommendations in this book are based on my experience as a medical herbalist, please know that I am not at odds with modern Western medicine. I work with all types of healers: medical doctors, acupuncturists, midwives, nurse practitioners, naturopaths, and other herbalists.

My abiding belief is that health care is really about the choices we make—not just what health plan or type of practitioner we choose, but the way we choose to live our lives outside the doctor's office. To me, taking the time to sit under a tree can be as important as the drugs you choose to take (or the herbs, for that matter). If adhering to an allopathic course of treatment for menopause makes you feel safe, I will not say you have chosen unwisely. On the contrary, my experience with women of all ages has shown me that—given the room, the chance, and the power to make their own informed, well-thought-out decisions—women usually choose the right path for themselves. My passion is to help women find their own authentic healing paths, which may mean suggesting a gentle tea for night sweats, a strong herbal regimen to help wean them off HRT, or helping a woman to find the best program including diet, herbs, and conventional medicine for osteoporosis, for example. Natural medicine is not in conflict or competition with standard medicine—at least not the type of herbalism I practice. If it is safe and effective, it's all just medicine. Closed-mindedness is our only true enemy. So please, feel free to show your health professional this book, but be prepared for a less-than-enthusiastic response from some doctors. If they can't support you in making your own informed decision, get a second opinion. It may take a little effort, but there are more physicians now who understand women's hesitancy to use conventional therapies for menopause, and some who are even eager to learn about alternative therapies.

This book is not meant for the coffee table. It is a self-help manual, which means it is to be used. If it gets stained with spilled tea or dog-eared by many hands, then I will consider the whole undertaking to have been worthwhile.

Finally, I am more than a decade older than when I wrote the first edition. Back then, I had been treating myself with food and herbal medicine after my own near-menopause due to extensive reproductive surgery at age twenty. I also based that first book on my first ten years in practice with women going through menopause—most with ease, some with great suffering. Now I have had another decade of clinical experience and my second thrilling opportunity to experience menopausal symptoms for myself. This time it is not "nearly menopause" but the real Change—absolutely final. I've listened more keenly to women who can't tolerate the taste of some herbs. After experimenting with one formula I developed in capsule form, I have five years of feedback from several hundred women. Thanks to all this Change for me, I aim in this edition for simplicity (fewer herbs per formula) and less paper (may more trees remain in the forests).

chapter 1

Perimenopause

Menopause occurs when the ovaries stop releasing eggs and menstruation ceases. The period of a woman's life called premenopause *can begin eight to ten years before complete menopause; it occurs when the normal monthly cycle of ovulation and menstruation becomes less regular. This entire period of transition is also known as* the climacteric *because the reproductive phase of life is reaching its climax. The formal term is perimenopause–literally, the time surrounding menopausal changes.*

The changes that accompany menopause are no less dramatic than those we experienced at puberty. Our bodies change, and with this comes new, strange feelings. The first part of this chapter discusses what is happening in the body at the cellular level. So that you can adapt to your own particular changes, the second part of the chapter provides practical, effective guidance that you can apply during the perimenopausal period and throughout this new stage of life.

THE REPRODUCTIVE PROCESS AND PERIMENOPAUSE

Our reproductive systems undergo natural, predictable changes from puberty to menopause. Each month, throughout the years between puberty and menopause, a woman's ovaries normally produce one egg, and the lining of the uterus thickens to prepare for a developing fetus should conception occur. If conception does not occur, this uterine lining (the endometrium) is discarded and released as menstrual blood.

Our endocrine systems produce hormones that circulate in our bodies and stimulate different functional activities at the cellular level. Estrogen, the hormone produced by the theca cells in the ovarian follicle, is key to the functions and changes in a woman's reproductive system. Women enter puberty when the body begins to produce significant levels of estrogen, and enter menopause when estrogen production declines.

When we are still having menstrual cycles, we are low in estrogen just before menstruation begins, especially on the first day. This is true whether you are twenty-two or forty-two. The brain senses low levels of estrogen circulating in the blood and sends a message to the pituitary gland in the brain to release *follicle-stimulating hormone* (FSH) into the bloodstream. FSH reaches the ovaries and stimulates development of an egg within its surrounding cavity (follicle). As the egg develops, the follicle makes estrogen, so levels in the bloodstream start to rise. This signals the brain that it can stop firing off such a strong message to the pituitary.

Meanwhile, back in the ovary, the developing egg keeps maturing while several others die off. The FSH decreases as the egg's secretion of estrogen signals the brain not to send so much FSH, but the FSH that is still being sent to the ovaries keeps the one egg growing, which ensures that the level of estrogen keeps rising for a time. The egg creates enough estrogen by about day fourteen to trigger a release of *luteinizing hormone* (LH) from the pituitary. LH causes more blood to circulate into the ovaries, bringing about two important changes. First, more cholesterol (a normal sterol found in the blood) is broken down in the ovaries and eventually changed into even more estrogen. A sterol is any one of a large group of plant or animal compounds related to both fats and alcohol. Second, enzymes help liberate the fully mature egg from its follicle for ovulation. The empty follicle now folds in on itself to form a soft lump, called the *corpus luteum* (yellow body)—it is yellow because of its fatty sterols, which are now made into a different female sex hormone: progesterone, the *pro-gestation* hormone that acts to prepare the uterus for implantation of the egg, to maintain pregnancy, and to promote milk production in the breasts. If there is no fertilization of the egg, the corpus luteum learns this through the chemistry of the blood. In turn, the corpus luteum stops making progesterone.

In perimenopause, there are fewer viable eggs than in past years and the ovaries become less responsive to FSH and LH. The hypothalamus in the brain sharply increases production of FSH and LH levels to stimulate the ovaries to produce estrogen. Some cycles never have enough estrogen built up for ovulation, although menstrual flow may still occur. Our bodies begin to need much less estrogen than was required for menstruation, conception, pregnancy, and lactation. But we do not completely lose all estrogen in menopause. If there is a healthy cushion of body fat, this provides raw material for estrogen production, and the adrenal glands also make a little. A lower level of estrogen may even have important advantages. As cycles become more irregular, estrogen-dependent symptoms such as painful cramps, tender breasts, menstrual migraines, and heavy bleeding from fibroids tend to improve. On the other hand, symptoms of low estrogen may potentially create new problems—at least until our bodies reach a new balance. Because estrogen is only one of many hormones whose levels are changing during this time, herbs that promote progesterone have also helped "low estrogen" symptoms of menopause, presumably by supporting our bodies in reaching that new balance.

THE ONSET OF PERIMENOPAUSE

Perimenopause is usually a gradual process, so women may not know exactly when it begins. If you are reasonably healthy and are older than thirty-six, a change from a fairly regular cycle to an irregular one may be an early sign of perimenopause.

Perimenopause commonly begins in the fifth decade of life but may start as early as the thirties or even the twenties. Menopause beginning in the twenties is not really menopause—it is premature ovarian failure. High-stress lifestyles, heightened economic and social worries, global pollution, a rise in gynecological surgeries, and other twenty-first-century factors may contribute to early onset of perimenopause, even among healthy women. It was thought until fairly recently that the earlier your first period (an event called the *menarche*) occurred, the earlier menopause was likely to occur. Now researchers are not certain.

Yet even if the experience of other women in your family turns out not to be an exact predictor of your age at menopause, talking with our elders about their histories can be invaluable. Our reproductive experiences are often similar. Listening to stories from mother, sisters, cousins, and aunts can encourage intimacy and a wealth of detail. Other factors to consider are personal health history, nutrition, ethnicity, climate, economic status, and social setting, all of which influence one another. For example, women who smoke or make a habit of eating fast food are more likely to have some degree of nutrient imbalance when menopause arrives, and therefore to have more severe symptoms such as hot flashes, depression, and dry skin. A history of health problems is associated with an earlier menopause. Health factors other than perimenopause can also make the menstrual cycle erratic—for example, traveling, illness, malnourishment, or rigorous athletic training. In this case, women may have unpredictable menstrual cycles, or more symptoms such as mood changes or hot flashes.

A NEW STAGE OF LIFE

For many women, perimenopause is a time of emotional ups and downs. Entering a new stage of life as well as coping with changing hormonal levels naturally make this a time for reevaluating life goals—assessing past accomplishments and defining or redefining the future.

You may wonder why, when you have been perfectly content with your beliefs up until now, you are suddenly questioning everything about your purpose in life and the way you have chosen to conduct it. And you may feel quite alone in your observations: You may feel you are the only one to notice that the weather is all wrong, that your favorite dish doesn't taste quite right. You catch your loved ones looking at you funny, which naturally makes you want to send them to summer camp, though they are far too old for that now. Meanwhile, you are worrying about aging, and on top of that, you have other challenges to face: family difficulties that tax your resources, career and financial choices to be assessed. When Tuesday's "I'm proud I did the best I could" clashes with Friday's "I've been on the planet for almost half a century and what have I got to show for it?"— stop and take a deep breath. These and myriad variations on having the emotional rug pulled out from under you are not necessarily signs of disease. Your mood swings could well be the opening stanza of perimenopause.

There is no healthy way to suppress strong emotions during this period. The best you can do is take a mental health break, even for five or ten minutes during a hectic schedule. Recognize your need for time to cool off, reflect, and get some space—and then find a way to do just that. By tuning in to what you are feeling, you will come to identify the known (and unknown) triggers that bring out these perhaps unwelcome feelings. Delve beneath the surface of your deeper unease. If you can take the time to muse on things until an insight rings true, you may even come to see the wisdom in this seeming madness. The process may be helped along with a relaxing cup of herb tea, a counseling session, or ten minutes locked in a bathroom stall breathing slowly and evenly. Perimenopause does not make women "crazy"; it makes us look inside. If we don't look inside, we will soon *feel* crazy. This is a time to deepen into your wisdom and begin to make the changes you have always wanted to make.

At any stage of perimenopause, the herbal self-care outlined in this chapter can help realign your essential, unchanging self with your emerging self. Less ideally, you can use megadoses of herbal supplements as natural drugs to "fix" a perimenopausal symptom, whether it is a mood change or an irregular cycle. The herb-as-drug approach can work for some women. But if we embrace the rite of passage that menopause is, we can take advantage of this special opportunity for deep transformation. Drugs, natural or pharmaceutical, are fine for short-term fixes, but, as you might guess, they have hidden costs, such as side effects needing still more treatment. Many of these are discussed in chapter 3.

The rest of this chapter explores common challenges faced during perimenopause. Some symptoms alarm women; some are more general signs of physical change you can observe in yourself. Still other challenges are nonphysical: emotional or mental self-doubts. All kinds of health changes may make a woman wonder whether she has entered menopause. Hot flashes, weight gain, and episodes of depression may occur in either perimenopause or menopause; these are covered in chapter 2.

MOOD SWINGS

When women speak of mood swings, they often mean depression, anxiety, or irritability, not upward swings of elation or joy. But you can experience both extremes under the biochemical influence of fluctuating hormones. If you want to fully experience your changing feelings without suppressing them or being run ragged by your emotions when they surface, try the nonaggressive herbal remedies in this section. The key to their effectiveness is consistency: Over time, these gentle herbal allies can help restore balance to your nervous system and hormonal cycle.

Whether a gentle herbal approach works depends on four factors: how long your stress level has driven your mood swings up and down, how troubling these emotional changes feel to you, how quickly or slowly your unique chemistry responds to the herbs, and what other steps you take to complement the healing herbs. As soon as all symptoms feel better or are almost gone (usually after two to three months), continue the same combination and dose for an extra three weeks, then reduce the dose by half for another three weeks. If you feel just as well after reducing the amount this way, simply keep a little extra on hand for future times when an occasional week back on the herbs will help you cope with a rough spell. If you should have any lingering symptoms after four or five months, continue taking the herbs at a half dose five days a week. When you feel ready, try reducing the dose again. Watch how well you respond, and skip the tea when your moods feel stable to you.

a note on measurements

Weight is always a more reliable measure in herbal medicine than size of container. In the case of dried herbs, you should use a simple kitchen scale to measure ounces by weight, not by volume. (Beakers are for liquid measurements.)

st. john's wort

Herbalists have used St. John's wort (*Hypericum perforatum*) for many years as a treatment for wound healing, diseases, or inflammation affecting nerves, and as a sedative, painkiller, and analgesic. Long before the term *depression* was coined, folk remedies that included St. John's wort were prescribed for common symptoms of depression, including insomnia, anxiety, and nervous unrest. In past decades, it has often appeared in European herb formulas for midlife women.

The herb combines anti-inflammatory, antiviral, and wound-healing properties with a restorative effect on the nerves. St. John's wort may reduce dependence on painkillers and antidepressants. Menopausal women on antidepressants should consult with an herbalist and their prescribing physician if they wish to include this herb in addition to, or in place of, their medication.

Contraindications: The popular and medical literature have devoted a lot of attention to the dangers of St. John's wort in terms of its interaction with other medications. It is always important to consult with a doctor or healthcare professional about drugs and any possible interactions with herbal remedies. But contrary to earlier reports, St. John's wort is not an SSRI (selective serotonin reuptake inhibitor), nor is it an MAOI (monoamine oxidase inhibitor). Unlike these two, and other pharmaceutical antidepressants, the exact mechanism of how St. John's wort improves mood is still unknown. There is no good scientific evidence that there is one active constituent responsible. The whole plant is the "active constituent."

Note: The often-repeated caution that St. John's wort cannot be taken with any antidepressant medications is now questioned, as some psychiatrists and herbalists working together to wean people off antidepressants use St. John's wort as well as other herbs as needed. Newer studies suggest St. John's wort compares favorably with the drug paroxetine, even in cases of moderate to severe depression.

Herbal Medicine

Concentrate for strengthening nerves

CONCENTRATED HERB EXTRACT	ACTIONS
½ oz. motherwort herb *(Leonurus cardiaca)*	Calms heart palpitations; bitter/cooling
½ oz. skullcap herb *(Scutellaria laterifolia)*	Reduces anxiety and tension headaches
1 oz. eleuthero root *(Eleutherococcus senticosus)*	Increases natural resistance to stress
2 oz. St. John's wort herb *(Hypericum perforatum)*	Lifts depression; repairs frayed nerves
2 oz. peppermint or spearmint leaf *(Mentha piperita, M. spicata)*	Cooling; helps liver functions; for flavor

Combine these herbal extracts. For sweet flavor, you can always add a pinch of stevia leaf, but it is strong, so a little goes a long way, especially the powdered and liquid products available. Take 1 teaspoon diluted in ¼ to 1 cup of water in the morning and evening. Take an additional dropperful every ten minutes as needed during stressful days or for better sleep at night. Use concentrate instead of tea for at least three hours before bedtime to avoid having to be awakened by a full bladder.

Five ounces will last five to fourteen days. Concentrated herb extracts are best stored in glass, not plastic, and away from direct sunlight or heat. They do not require refrigeration. A dark brown or blue glass bottle available from some drugstores and many online suppliers (see Resources) allows the herb formula to sit where it will be remembered, perhaps the cupboard of glasses and cups that you open every day. The main point is that herbs are best stored in a cool, dry, place. For chronic stress, expect to take for a minimum of two months before experiencing lasting benefits. For the best effect, take the full dosage over six months and then half-strength for another four months.

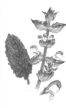

Tea for strengthening nerves

DRIED HERBS	ACTIONS
2 oz. skullcap herb (*Scutellaria laterifolia*)	Reduces anxiety; relieves tension headaches
4 oz. lemon balm leaf (*Melissa officinalis*)	Lifts depression; good for immunity, taste
1 oz. passionflower vine (*Passiflora incarnata*)	Lessens physical and emotional pain
1 oz. chamomile flower (*Matricaria recutita*)	Calms effects of stress on digestion

Cover ½ ounce of the herb tea blend with 3½ cups of boiling water in a teapot or container with a well-fitting lid. Let stand for fifteen minutes before straining. Drink 1 cup, hot or cold, three times a day. If you prefer, sip tea throughout the day or drink two larger glasses twice a day. You can add stevia or agave syrup to taste.

Eight ounces of dried herb will last two weeks if used daily at this dose.

Nutrition

Review the following suggestions for whole foods that provide vitamins and minerals to address your mood, as well as the list of natural supplements.

wise food choices

- Choose foods high in vitamin C: red, green, yellow bell peppers; fresh broccoli; citrus fruits; rosehip jam (although vitamin C is lost in cooking except in some high-quality brands, natural fruit pectins and bioflavonoids offer other benefits); baked potatoes.

- For healthy nerves, eat foods high in B vitamin complex: dark green leafy vegetables and whole grains such as brown rice, polenta, buckwheat, whole wheat with bran, and wheat germ.

- Eat one clove of raw or lightly steamed garlic in food daily to protect the heart from long-term stress. Fresh garlic provides zinc, chromium, and other nutrients, and it kills off microbes. Cooked garlic and deodorized garlic capsules benefit the heart but have fewer immune benefits. Aged garlic extracts have also been shown by medical research to reduce cancer risk. For all these reasons, adding some form of garlic in a mix of whole foods on a daily or weekly basis is an all-around beneficial practice.

- Reduce animal fats and excess protein. Calcium from dairy foods and iron from meat is not well used when a woman is under chronic stress, so eating more doesn't add energy.

- Replace chicken or red meat with tofu, tempeh, or other soy protein one or two times a week.

❀ Occasionally add 1 teaspoon to 1 tablespoon sesame seeds or tahini (the delicious paste of ground sesame seeds) to salads; use tahini on crackers instead of margarine or butter. For a vegetable dip or satisfying nondairy sandwich spread, mix ⅓ cup tahini with 1 tablespoon water and 1 to 2 teaspoons miso (rice, barley, or soybean paste) to taste with a spoon, fork, or whisk, until smooth and creamy. Sesame seeds are high in calcium and other nutrients, and the oil provides essential fatty acids; though women concerned with weight gain and heart health are well advised to lower dietary fats, we all require some healthy oils for good nerve function and immunity. When we feel nourished and eat small amounts of these concentrated, healthy plant oils, our craving for inappropriate fats lessens. For those who are interested, the use of sesame seed has ancient spiritual reverberations associated with physical protection.

supplements

❀ Vitamin A, beta-carotene

❀ Vitamin B complex

❀ Vitamin C

❀ Folic acid

❀ Balanced calcium and magnesium (see "Osteoporosis" in chapter 2)

❀ Deodorized garlic capsules as directed on labels if you prefer them to steamed or raw garlic in food

In Addition

❀ Occasionally work in the garden for half an hour (if you already enjoy gardening, you know that a half hour can stretch into hours because getting your hands in the dirt is so relaxing and weeding gets out so much tension).

❀ Stretch for ten minutes on the floor before crawling into bed.

❀ Take four drops of Tiger Lily flower essence (available from the Flower Essence Society; see Resources) four times a day, or use it in your bathwater for added relaxation. Flower essences are not essential oils such as lavender or peppermint. Essences are water-based remedies that belong to the discipline of Vibrational Medicine.

❀ Make a huge, double-strength batch of hot chamomile tea (4 to 8 ounces of herb in 1 to 2 quarts of water); strain and reserve 1 cup for sipping, adding a little honey if you wish. Pour the rest into a hot bath. Light a candle, turn off the lights, and relax for at least fifteen minutes. Alternatively, mix four to eight drops of chamomile or lavender essential oil into a tub of water and soak away the tension of the day.

❀ Only have a shower? Put three drops of any relaxing essential oil on a washcloth; holding it under the stream of water about 10 inches from your face, gently breathe in the steam. Then wash your body with this lightly scented cloth instead of soap.

ERRATIC MENSTRUAL CYCLES

As you enter perimenopause, you may experience erratic menstrual cycles. Menstrual periods continue as long as the ovaries secrete some estrogen, because the hormone builds up the uterine lining, which later leaves the body as menstrual blood. Meanwhile, your body is adjusting to its new hormonal balance in the following way. Most of the eggs your ovaries contained at birth have been used by now, one way or another, either leading to a pregnancy or washed out in a menstrual flow. Some have naturally died off with each ovulation. A few viable eggs may still be present at this point, but ovulation is erratic. If an egg is not developing, there is no ovulation. Without ovulation, there is a drop in progesterone, which is even more significant than the drop in estrogen. For a while during perimenopause it can be normal to have a higher level of both FSH and LH in the blood, but without enough progesterone, the pituitary gland in the brain sends out less and less LH. Why? Perhaps the pituitary knows better than to keep on trying to stimulate an egg to develop in a follicle if it senses biochemically that the egg is not there. The lack of this ovarian hormone is what informs "headquarters" in the pituitary. Just to be sure, the FSH from the brain takes up the slack by increasing its level in the bloodstream, to get at least some response, if possible, out of the ovaries. Eventually, FSH production runs out, too. This may be why herbs that seem to promote progesterone are as important for helping to normalize an erratic perimenopausal cycle as herbs that seem to promote estrogen. Fortunately, these herbs are not as strong as pharmaceutical replacement hormones, so they tend to promote only those levels of hormones that the body is capable of utilizing in a healthy way.

Herbs with progestational or estrogenic effects often regulate an erratic cycle. With their assistance, you need not experience extreme irregularities or sudden heavy bleeding that can lead to embarrassing situations when you thought you were all done with menstruation. Nor does the transition have to be so irregular that it sends you into a panic over missed periods suggesting a possibly unwanted pregnancy. But herbs cannot work against nature. No vegetable matter on this planet can put an egg back in an ovary for fertilization. Nor can any healing plant force the uterine lining to build up and flow out again after a woman is past her time for menstruation. That said, there are many documented cases of women who have not menstruated for a year or longer and then taken hormonally active herbs, only to have their menstrual flow resume. Sometimes this was desirable, sometimes not. Rather than overstimulating the uterus, the herbs may have been acting as subtle biological nutrition for a woman with some remaining egg follicles and borderline hormone levels. In this case, the hormonal herbs simply allowed the uterine lining that had built up over time without monthly release to be cleared out in a few unanticipated menstrual flows. Though most women in perimenopause are functionally infertile (eggs present, implantation unlikely), women choosing herbs for improved health need to be aware that irregular flows always carry a risk of pregnancy.

If you are new to the world of herbs, you should know that there is no reason to be afraid of the following herb teas. They will not cause dangerous postmenopausal bleeding. Medicinal plants are powerful, but unlike poisonous plants or pharmaceutical drugs, these herbs are subject to the body's own healthy self-regulation. Medicinal herb constituents are recommended and usually ingested in lower doses than are isolated chemicals. Even capsules, teas, tinctures, and concentrated extracts are unprocessed natural products compared to prescription drugs. The body recognizes plant starches, aromatic oils, and the like, which break down in normal metabolism. The body has sophisticated pathways for speeding the clearance of nutrients with physiological effects, as a part of the design for dynamic homeostasis (active state of health). These pathways range from making herb chemicals more water-soluble for easier excretion to binding them with liver proteins while stimulating intestinal activity. Herb scientists are beginning to ask if herb chemistry is less important than understanding the complex web of how each whole person's enzymes, heartbeat, and mood co-determine how, why, and when herbs work. This could explain why past research based on isolated herb chemicals is often overturned by new studies.

Herbal Medicine

Concentrate for erratic cycles

CONCENTRATED HERB EXTRACT

4 oz. chaste berry seed (*Vitex agnus-castus*)

2 oz. lady's mantle herb (*Alchemilla vulgaris*)

2 oz. nettle leaf (*Urtica dioica*)

ACTIONS

Promotes pituitary control over timing of cycle

Relaxing reproductive tonic

Provides minerals and nutrition to all cells

Combine these herbal extracts. Take 1 teaspoon in 1 cup of water in the morning and evening, from the first day without an active flow through to the next premenstrual phase. Then, skip this until the next end of the period. In ninety days or so (which may or may not include three periods), the cycle will begin to be more predictable. At this stage, take the herbs only once a day; morning is best.

Eight ounces will last about three weeks.

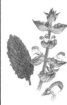

Tea for erratic cycles

DRIED HERBS	ACTIONS
4 oz. chaste berry seed *(Vitex agnus-castus)*	Promotes pituitary control over timing of cycle
2 oz. lady's mantle herb *(Alchemilla vulgaris)*	Relaxing reproductive tonic
2 oz. rosemary leaf *(Rosmarinus officinalis)*	Aids digestion; for flavor

Add ½ ounce of the mixture to 3½ cups of boiling water in a teapot or container with a well-fitting lid. Let stand for fifteen minutes before straining. Drink 1 cup hot or cold, depending on the season and your preference, up to three times a day.

Eight ounces will last two weeks or longer.

Nutrition

Review the following suggestions for whole foods that provide vitamins and minerals to address erratic menstrual cycles, as well as the list of natural supplements.

wise food choices

❀ Avoid fats, especially heated oils and animal fats such as those in cheese and red meat.

❀ Avoid excess protein, packaged convenience foods, refined flour, sugar, and junk food.

❀ Eat three carrots or drink 10 ounces of fresh carrot juice daily for a week before you expect your flow to begin, even if that part of the monthly cycle is early or late.

❀ Eat sweet potatoes, yams, or baked organic potatoes (your choice) three times a week.

❀ Add ½ to 1 teaspoon or even just a sprinkling of fennel seeds to Italian or East Indian sauces and dishes, such as rice pilaf or polenta with sun-dried tomatoes.

❀ Eat salads with cucumber, chopped onion, dill, and lemon juice, to taste.

supplements

❀ Evening primrose oil. Because capsules may vary in milligrams, the dose is actually a range. A minimum dose—six to ten capsules daily of 500 milligrams each or more—is expensive, but this supplement may be needed only for six weeks or so, making it more practical and affordable. Also, borage and black currant oil are cheaper sources of GLA (gamma-linoleic acid), but effects vary, so follow recommended dosages on labels.

❀ Home-sprouted seeds and legumes of every kind cost only pennies a day and are a great alternative to evening primrose oil. Sprouted seeds and raw nuts provide easily digested plant protein and good-quality essential fatty acids in a water-based form we can handle, in addition to enzymes helpful to good metabolism.

In Addition

❀ Try the Ten-Minute Visualization (see page 20).

SPOTTING AND FLOODING

During perimenopause, you may notice that the time between periods is shorter, but the flow is less than in the past. These spotty periods may alternate with normal cycles or be replaced by sudden, gushing flow (flooding) for five to eight days. In itself, heavy blood loss isn't abnormal, but it is wise to have a trusted health-care provider rule out other causes, such as fibroids or malignancy. More than two "normal" pads in thirty minutes is a hemorrhage. Three or four extremely heavy flows in a row can cause anemia. Even if anemia is only temporary, you can follow the recommendations below to correct or prevent it. If you lose a lot more blood than you normally do each month, pay attention to other signs of anemia, such as a pale tongue and inner edges of eyelids, fatigue, cold hands and feet, shallow breathing, or noticing that minor cuts and wounds take a longer than normal time to heal.

Herbal Medicine

Concentrate for heavy bleeding

CONCENTRATED HERB EXTRACT

4 oz. nettle leaf (*Urtica dioica*)

1 oz. angelica root (*Angelica archangelica*, not dong quai–a different species, *A. sinensis*)

1 oz. lady's mantle herb (*Alchemilla vulgaris*)

ACTIONS

Mineral-rich antihemorrhagic

Warms and moves blood; improves immune "tone" in Chinese medicine

Astringent; calming; uterine tonic

Combine these herbal extracts. Take 1 teaspoon in 1 cup of water in the morning and evening. Take an extra dropperful every ten minutes until excess bleeding slows or stops.

Six ounces will last ten days.

Note: *All vaginal bleeding that does not respond to herbs within three days is best diagnosed by a licensed practitioner before continuing self-care at home. Rest often with legs up, and keep drinking fluids.*

Ten-Minute Visualization

Don't just read this—try it, trusting in your body's ancient wisdom to benefit from this and every effort you make to bring healing from within. Perhaps you could make a tape of yourself speaking the following words and listen to them every day. If you record the visualization, you may wish to leave a silent pause of thirty seconds or more where asterisks (*) appear. Routinely practicing this visualization allows your whole spirit, mind, and body to reset your biological clock gently but firmly over a twenty-eight-day lunar cycle. You may also use this visualization whenever you need to get centered. Begin by sitting comfortably, in a quiet, dark space, if possible.

Breathe deeply, exhaling all your thoughts and worries. Breathe in. Let it all go while you straighten your spine. On your next in-breath, count to three. * Count to three as you breathe out. * Repeat this for the next few minutes, for a total of twenty-one times. * Count to four as you breathe in. * Count to four as you breathe out. * Repeat this once. * Allow your breathing to continue evenly and slowly, in and out. In and out. You are sitting in perfect balance in a comfortable darkness. Continue to breathe evenly and slowly. *

With every in-breath, the darkness fades up to a deep and lovely blue. With every out-breath, the sky fills slowly with light, until you can see the whole Earth from where you sit. Breathe in and out. * Watch your breathing seem to draw the sun as it appears over the horizon. Breathe it down into the sea at sunset. Breathe in and out seven times in stillness and peace.

With your next in-breath, see the moon rise over the Earth's horizon. Breathe in evenly, breathe out slowly so the moon can glide up effortlessly. * When the moon is at its highest so the moonbeams splash down on you, it will start to set. When its silver-violet light has entirely disappeared, breathe in and out in comfortable darkness seven times. Then you will know it is time to gently open your eyes. *

There is something about this "time-out" that seems to create a sense of having more time. Each time you follow this exercise for aligning with your natural timing, you will be using your own creative impulse to gain in health and inner peace.

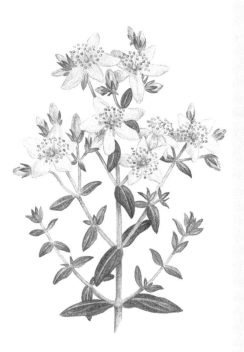

Tea for heavy bleeding

DRIED HERBS	ACTIONS
2 oz. lady's mantle herb (*Alchemilla vulgaris*)	Tones bleeding uterine walls; balances and calms
1 oz. raspberry leaf (*Rubus idaeus*)	Slows blood loss; replaces lost fluid and calcium
2 oz. nettle leaf (*Urtica dioica*)	Replaces lost fluids; rich in minerals, vitamins
2 oz. rosehips (*Rosa canina*)	Vitamin C for iron, mineral assimilation; for taste
½ oz. rose flowers (*Rosa* species)	Organically grown buds or petals reduce bleeding, infection
½ oz. sage leaf (*Salvia officinalis*)	Hormone balancing; astringent; aids digestion

Add ½ ounce of the mixture to 3½ cups of boiling water in a teapot or container with a well-fitting lid. Let stand for fifteen minutes before straining. Drink 1 cup, hot or cold, three times a day. You may sip tea throughout the day or drink two larger glasses twice a day, but be sure you drink 3 cups a day.

Six ounces will last thirty days.

Nutrition

Review the following suggestions for whole foods that provide vitamins and minerals to address heavy bleeding.

wise food choices

Occasional heavy blood loss or prolonged spotting can lead to anemia. To prevent anemia, obtain iron from these food sources, which won't cause constipation as supplements often do:

* Eat unsulfured dried apricots soaked for fifteen minutes or longer in water.
* Eat ten raw pumpkin seeds a day on salads or as a quick-energy snack.
* Drizzle 1 tablespoon blackstrap molasses over old-fashioned (not microwaved or instant) oatmeal on cold mornings.
* Sprinkle one-eighth teaspoon cinnamon on applesauce on warm mornings or for late-night snacks instead of sweets or bread.
* Eat red, yellow, and green vegetables, especially steamed kale and spinach.
* Eat root vegetables: burdock chopped like carrots in soup, grated beets or jicama in salads.
* Add nasturtium flowers and leaves and watercress to salads.

❋ A dash of red cayenne pepper to taste whenever practical in salad dressing, on grains, or in soups. This may bring symptoms of heat (hot flashes, night sweats) for some women. If this happens, you may prefer to discontinue cayenne in favor of other recommendations here for spotting or bleeding.

Alternatively, for short-term effects against spotting and bleeding, mix ¼ teaspoon cayenne powder in 2 teaspoons honey; knock back quickly, with a chaser of water, tomato juice, or some other juice you like, four times a day for one to three days, or until flooding stops. This remedy will *not* burn the stomach, even though initially it may feel like it! To avoid the use of honey, take ¼ teaspoon cayenne powder wrapped in edible starch papers, available at natural-food stores, or take the pepper in capsule (though these are less reliable), 6 "00" size, four times a day with water, juice, or a piece of plain bread to assist digestion. If you do not see any benefits in a few hours to one day, check with your health-care provider.

In Addition

❋ Rest frequently during spotting or flooding. Raise the legs and feet on a few pillows above the head and heart.

❋ Every night for a week, take a bath (not too hot) containing five drops each any or all three of these essential oils: chamomile, lavender, clary sage.

❋ Sell your television and watch clouds instead (better plots).

❋ Excuse yourself from work for an hour or two ("Something has come up") or leave a friendly but clear message on your phone indicating that you are in a conference or otherwise occupied and unavailable. Then go talk with your guardian angels for an hour. After that, you can catch up on any urgent tasks or pleasant projects with your mind and body renewed.

IMPROVING FERTILITY

You may find yourself entering perimenopause and experiencing a reduction in fertility but still wanting to have a child. Although there is a popular belief that having a baby later in life entails unacceptable health risks, there is no real reason to assume that a healthy forty-year-old, for example, is "lucky" to experience a normal pregnancy. Recent studies indicate that the increase in Down syndrome babies born to women over forty, though reliably documented, is not necessarily due to the age of the ovum. At age forty, chances are one in a hundred that a mother will give birth to a Down child, but conversely, that also means the child will be normal ninety-nine times out of a hundred. Other theories suggest that the age of male partners, frequency of intercourse, and external cofactors such as X-rays, environmental toxins, and illness may play a role in the incidence of Down syndrome.

Today, plenty of noninvasive support is available to women who face declining fertility but want to have a child. Women who are wise in the ways of herbal medicine have known for millennia which plants are best for restoring natural functions. A first blessing on your intention to conceive is to take the following combination of herbal extracts. A second blessing comes with each simple cup of womb-honoring herbal tea. During menstruation, skip the extract but continue with the herbal tea. If conception occurs, continue with the tea only.

In general, use the following combinations for a minimum of three months. You can safely take these herbs for up to five years, although most women will need them for only one to two years. If you take them for more than two years, skip the regimen one day a week to give your body a rest.

If you feel a deep need to be important in the life of a child, and natural pregnancy is not possible for you, by all means work to find alternative ways to "mother." Many, many women consider life without children to provide other riches; some women teach their own special skills to children in community groups, and others adopt or offer loving homes as foster parents to children who desperately need them. Seek and you will find your own special way.

Herbal Medicine

Concentrate for improving fertility

CONCENTRATED HERB EXTRACT	ACTIONS
4 oz. chaste berry seed (*Vitex agnus-castus*)	Promotes conception
4 oz. raspberry leaf (*Rubus idaeus*)	Nourishing uterine tonic; calcium-rich; calming

Combine these herbal extracts. Take 1 teaspoon in 1 cup of water twice per day, in the morning and evening.

Eight ounces will last approximately three weeks.

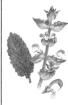

Tea for improving fertility

DRIED HERBS	ACTIONS
2 oz. Jamaican sarsaparilla root (*Smilax ornata*)	Balances hormones; cleanses skin; supports lymph, immunity
2 oz. raspberry leaf (*Rubus idaeus*)	Nourishing tonic; provides calcium
1 oz. red clover flower (*Trifolium pratense*)	Promotes estrogenic balance and fertility
1½ oz. rosehips (*Rosa canina*)	Bioflavonoids promote tissue repair
1½ oz. hibiscus flower (*Hibiscus sabdariffa*)	Bioflavonoids support kidneys and circulation

Add ½ ounce of the mixture to 3½ cups of boiling water in a teapot or other container with a tight-fitting lid. Let stand for fifteen minutes before straining. Drink 1 cup, hot or cold, one to three times per day. At a minimum, drink 1 cup a day for ninety days before reassessing. Eight ounces will last approximately two weeks.

Nutrition

Review the following suggestions for whole foods that provide vitamins and minerals to improve fertility, as well as the list of natural supplements.

wise food choices

- ❀ Eat watermelon, pomegranates, fresh figs, and other fruit with seeds, all in season.

- ❀ Eat zucchini, squash, or other vegetables, in soup or stir-fried.

- ❀ Try live green sprouts, such as alfalfa, sunflower, aduki, lentil, fenugreek, and onion.

- ❀ Try "wild weed" salads: dandelion, mustard greens, nettle shoots, lamb's quarters, miner's lettuce, wild lettuce, and edible Chinese chrysanthemums.

- ❀ Make homemade nondairy pesto with basil, thyme, olive oil, powdered dulse or kelp, and fresh nuts.

- ❀ Eat one freshly cracked walnut per day.

- ❀ Sprinkle one to 3 teaspoons coarsely chopped raw seeds or nuts on salads, three times per week.

- ❀ Eat soy beans, other soy foods (such as tofu or tempeh), or 1 tablespoon soy flour mixed with other flours, two to five times per week.

- ❀ Make curried dal (lentils) with garlic, cumin, turmeric, mild or hot to taste.

* For nonvegans and nonvegetarians, eat two eggs, or 4 ounces lean white fish, or 3 ounces cooked lamb, once a week.

* Avoid any foods that trigger allergies.

Even though our bodies are quite capable of thriving on a vegetarian diet, there is no getting around the fact that the sterols provided by meat consumption are stimulating to the human endocrine system. Organic animal fats and proteins in moderation can help weak, stressed, or underweight women. (Unfortunately, commercial hormones added to butter, eggs, meat, and cheese make many women feel worse.) To replace this animal energy, vegetarians and vegans need to emphasize the more concentrated plant protein foods in the other categories just suggested.

supplements

* Folic acid

* Vitamin D from natural sunlight (about twenty minutes per day)

Your body naturally synthesizes vitamin D when you allow sunshine to fall on your skin, unprotected by sunscreen. This does not mean tanning salons or risking skin cancer at the beach. Taking a ten- to twenty-minute walk (but not during the peak hours of 10 AM to 2 PM) is an excellent way to supplement vitamin D as well as give yourself some pleasant exercise, which prevents osteoporosis and reduces stress or tension in the body. Of course, supplementing with vitamin D has well-known advantages, covered elsewhere.

In Addition

* To 1 ounce sweet almond oil, add twenty-one drops essential oil of jasmine. Massage the abdomen, breasts, and underarms. For the full treatment worthy of any goddess, occasionally spend one to two hours massaging and soothing tired skin, paying special attention to sore spots as well as stretching and kneading the muscles in the calves, thighs, forearms, and fingers. Perhaps have someone else rub your back, neck, and shoulders.

* Castor oil packs (see page 26) placed over the abdomen or lower back once or twice a week can help the body self-repair if old scars are blocking conception. The messiness of these packs is worth the cleanup, especially when you consider the bonus of great pelvic circulation.

* Yoga will open the pelvis, as well as prepare ligaments and muscles for the possibility of pregnancy.

* Create a secret ceremony, known only to you and your lover, to create a receptive mood, to protect the rich bloom of your passion, and to open both of you to the sacred gift of a child.

* Visualizing healthy change and conception has great power here. Many women who are now mothers of healthy children were told that their sonograms or other tests ruled out any reasonable expectation of conception. This is a good time for women to move beyond "reason"

to the miracle. We know that our emotions affect our hormones, and that our hormones affect our fertility. Having lost our conscious connection to the body's ways doesn't mean we have lost our subconscious connection to dream, vision, purpose, or love.

castor oil pack

Castor oil, made from the castor bean plant (*Ricinus communis*, also called Palma Christi in folklore), can be used externally in a hot compress to reduce swelling and overgrowths of fibrous tissue. It is available at herb shops, natural-food stores, and some drugstores, as well as from many of the suppliers listed in the Resources section.

Heat at least 4 ounces of castor oil in a small saucepan or a double boiler. The oil is the right temperature when a drop on your wrist is hot but not uncomfortably so. To avoid burns and grease fires, take special care not to spill the oil. Pour the oil into the center of a hand towel or large piece of flannel and fold the fabric over once or twice to contain the oil. Add more oil as needed to saturate the fabric. Place the warm, oily cloth on the skin over the lower abdomen or lower back. Lay a hot-water bottle or another clean, dry towel over the oil-soaked towel to reduce heat loss. Leave it on your skin for twenty minutes to an hour—as long as it remains warm (the hot-water bottle can be refilled as needed, and you can add fresh, heated castor oil).

Repeat no more than twice a week for severe conditions—the breakdown of tissue should not proceed faster than the body's ability to safely eliminate what is being stirred up. Increased blood flow from the hot oil pack improves general circulation and elimination. It can also help heal any bruise, swelling, or growth.

Adding therapeutically fragrant, spiritually uplifting essential oils (not chemical perfumes) is especially helpful when stress or depression about self-image accompany infertility, fibroids, and other reproductive conditions. These are added to the castor oil not while it is heating—the essential (volatile) oils would evaporate—but just before you pour it into the towel. For every 3 to 5 ounces of warm castor oil, add three or four drops each of one or more of the following pure essential oils (available at herb or natural-food stores, or by mail order—see Resources): geranium, marjoram, clary sage, ginger. They are expensive, but small amounts last a long time.

SEXUALITY AND VAGINAL CHANGES

You may notice some of the following physical changes as your estrogen levels decline during perimenopause; all of them are perfectly normal and healthy. The fat cushion in the labia is reabsorbed, the smaller lips (labia minora) may eventually disappear, the vaginal canal gets a little smaller, the vaginal wall becomes thinner. The cells of the vaginal walls are also less cornified (less tough, which means more sensitive to both pleasant pressure and potential irritation). The crevice where the top of the vagina folds in on itself to become the cervix gets a little shallower. The size of the cervix also decreases, and the glands in the mucous membrane surfaces throughout the vaginal canal secrete lubricants less actively.

These effects of decreasing estrogen happen over time and vary in degree from woman to woman. But don't believe for a minute that good sex disappears in tandem with these changes. Many postmenopausal women in their sixties and seventies have reported satisfying sex, good lubrication, low incidences of infection, and an abundant well of desire. For many of us, lubrication must now be stimulated by great loving, not just any old hormonal flush of youth. It may take longer to bring the bucket to the top of the well, but, as they say, the water tastes sweeter because it rises from so deep. That thirst is one you can choose to either let grow or ignore if there is no lover worthy of your bed. With no fear of pregnancy to put a crimp in your pleasure, you may know full body ecstasy now, even if you haven't known it before.

The following combination nourishes the sex drive when it is used in small doses over time. This tones the reproductive tissues to optimize sensuality.

Herbal Medicine

Concentrate for libido

CONCENTRATED HERB EXTRACT

4 oz. shatavari *(Asparagus racemosa)*

3½ oz. maca root *(Lepidium meyenii)*

½ oz. licorice root *(Glycyrrhiza glabra)*

ACTIONS

East Indian herb; increases lubrication

South American food and tonic for sex drive

Moistening; lessens inflammation; helps immunity

Combine these herbal extracts. Take 1 teaspoon in 1 cup of water in the morning and evening. Eight ounces will last thirty days.

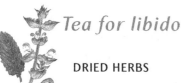

Tea for libido

DRIED HERBS	ACTIONS
3½ oz. shatavari *(Asparagus racemosa)*	East Indian herb; increases lubrication
3½ oz. maca root *(Lepidium meyenii)*	South American food and tonic for sex drive
½ oz. licorice root *(Glycyrrhiza glabra)*	Moistening; lessens inflammation; helps immunity
½ oz. organically grown rose petals *(Rosa species)*	Lessens bleeding, infection

Add ½ ounce of the mixture to 3½ cups of boiling water in a teapot or container with a well-fitting lid. Let the herb blend steep in the water, covered, for fifteen minutes before straining. Drink 1 cup, hot or cold, up to three times a day.

Note: *The rose petals must be organic; leave them out if you do not have a reliable source. If you dislike the flavor or are sensitive to licorice, leave that out.*

Eight ounces will last about three weeks.

Nutrition

Review the following suggestions for whole foods that provide vitamins and minerals to address sexuality and vaginal changes, as well as the list of natural supplements.

wise food choices

❀ Avoid excess coffee and alcohol.

❀ Soy foods, sprouted lentils, raw snow peas, and cooked green peas naturally increase your level of estrogen; use these according to your personal taste. For a discussion of the effects of these foods, see the nutrition section in "Hot Flashes and Night Sweats" in chapter 2.

❀ Add borage flowers, violet flowers, cucumber slices, and basil leaves in season to salads and sandwiches.

supplements

❀ Flaxseeds, 1 teaspoon daily. Soak in water for twenty minutes; add to blended fruit drinks and salad dressings, or stir into cooked grains shortly before serving. You can also stir 1 to 2 teaspoons of ground seeds into one or two glasses of water and drink the mixture immediately before or between meals. Refrigerate flaxseeds and grind them fresh, otherwise they will quickly become rancid. Also, if you don't drink the mixture immediately, it will become jelly-like, a rather unpleasant texture for drinking. Or, if you prefer, take capsules as directed on labels.

❀ Vitamin E, 200 to 300 I.U. (international units) three times a day. After a week, reduce the amount to 400 I.U. daily. More is not always better—don't take more than 1,200 I.U. daily. If you have diabetes, hypertension, or a rheumatic heart condition, don't use more than 100 I.U. daily. Studies show all types of vitamin E may provide benefit, but if possible, choose mixed natural tocopherols.

❀ Vitamin C, 1 gram three times a day, preferably with meals and your vitamin E doses.

In Addition

❀ Use essential oils with a reputation for aphrodisiac qualities as bath or massage oils. The use of lubricating aromatherapy for the vagina can help you get in touch with your body. A favorite combination is vitamin E oil blended with essential (volatile) oil of sandalwood, ylang ylang, or clary sage. To make your own massage or bath blend, place a total of nine drops of one or all of the above essential oils in ½ ounce of vitamin E oil and ½ ounce of sesame, almond, or any other unheated vegetable oil. Stir ¼ teaspoon into a bath or apply a few drops of the blend to fingertips; massage skin and genitalia. Lubricating herb mixtures shouldn't sting or irritate; don't use when skin is broken. If the oil does cause redness, you may have too strong a blend; try adding more vitamin E or vegetable oil. Also, rinse with plain cold water and wait a few days before trying again.

❀ Practice pelvic floor exercises (see page 31) five minutes a day to strengthen the muscles that make up the pelvic floor.

❀ Sex stimulates secretion of moisture and germ-fighting enzymes in the mucous membranes of vaginal walls. If you experience discomfort in intercourse, or if vaginal dryness persists despite desire, your vagina may have an infection or the membranes may be thinning. For a fuller discussion of vaginal problems, see "Vaginal Thinning and Dryness" in chapter 2.

❀ Don't douche much or at all. Among other things, it dries the vagina's mucous membranes, setting the scene for future irritation or infection. If you want to douche on occasion for relief of symptoms or for other reasons, follow the directions below.

To clear an itchy yeast infection or replenish vaginal membranes after repeated or severe vaginal infections, herbalists prefer to soothe and moisturize with herbally medicated suppositories extracted in an oil base. Companies offering these are listed in Resources. If used as directed here, women may find relief from one-time rinsing (not douching) with toning and healing herbs such as lady's mantle, chamomile, sage, and licorice. Cover 1 ounce of any one or two (not all) with a pint of boiling water. After letting the mixture stand for fifteen minutes, strain and cool to a comfortable body temperature, and fill a douche bag with a simple bulb and applicator from the drugstore. Insert the applicator tube into just the first inch or two of the vaginal opening and gently squeeze the bulb to introduce the liquid only into the outer vaginal canal. Or, if you do not have a douche bag, pour the mixture as a rinse over the vaginal folds while holding them open with the clean fingers of one hand. Douche no more than three days in a row and only if needed. After chronic infections, you can repeat the treatment every two weeks to help restore the integrity of the vaginal walls.

For a fuller discussion of douching, see "Vaginal Thinning and Dryness" in chapter 2.

❀ You can use herbal oils (not the same as essential or volatile oils) as frequently as needed. They help during intercourse to lubricate vaginal tissues, but they do more than reduce friction. St. John's wort and wild yam herb oils can lessen inflammation, heal raw places on the vaginal wall or cervix, and even be absorbed for mild local hormonal benefits. These can be purchased, but some are more expensive than they need to be. If you are willing to fool around in the kitchen for two or three hours, you can make your own milder but effective, affordable vaginal salve or cream (see "Nourishing Herbal Salve for Vaginal Comfort" on page 32).

WHOLE-BODY EFFECTS OF PERIMENOPAUSE

Whenever signs and symptoms of pre- or perimenopause are complicated or severe enough to demand professional attention, the cause may be a hormonal imbalance unrelated to estrogen or progesterone. Hormonal levels may fluctuate from the way the pancreas controls blood sugar, the adrenal glands' response to stress and immunity, thyroid changes affecting metabolism, and complex endocrine effects on sleep, mood, and the state of your nerves. To give just one example, several "menopausal" symptoms—such as moodiness, weight gain, low energy, and change in cycle—could be attributed just as well to undiagnosed hypothyroidism; that is, low thyroid function.

The possibilities can seem discouraging to sort out, so if you don't know whether your periods and moods are changing because of menopause or a medical condition, see a nurse-practitioner, midwife, or other experienced female health-care provider, and talk with other women. If it's your style, read the relevant paragraphs in a dictionary of symptoms. Use the Internet with caution; it's a vector of both medical misinformation and life-saving help. Weight gain, changes in skin texture, unexpected desires—all have a few common causes. But don't blindly accept the opinions of others regarding causes and a diagnosis if they do not ring true. You know yourself better than anyone else, and you are the person who can best know how to balance your body's systems.

To achieve balance within, you will need to experiment and try some different herbal combinations. Although it may seem an odd comparison, the process is much like balancing a tire on a car. As every woman who has changed a tire knows, each of the lug nuts (four huge bolts) must be tightened only a little at a time, but not in logical progression around the wheel. If you completely tighten a bolt before going on to the next, by the time all four are tightened, the wheel will have twisted just enough to be off balance. We must do a little here, a little there, switching back and forth, not necessarily in logical order, turning the bolts a little more, until every bolt in the circle can be tightened with just one more turn of the wrench. The properly balanced wheel rolls smoothly along the ground without wobbling.

pelvic floor exercises

Formerly known as kegels, these exercises cost no money and require no classes. Even a few weeks of practice makes a difference. Like yoga, the more consistently and the more slowly you do these painless exercises, the better the effects. Pelvic floor exercises are very safe and help most women. Among other benefits, they reduce pelvic organ prolapse in a mother who has borderline muscle tone. More universal is their effect on bladder and vaginal tone, helping women with urinary incontinence. If you cannot hold urine when you laugh, sneeze, strain, or jump up and down, you need to do pelvic floor exercises.

Pelvic floor exercises strengthen the muscles that make up the pelvic "floor" and add good blood flow. The pelvis is like a big basin or fruit bowl, with openings at the bottom that we control through muscle tone. Two pairs of symmetrical muscles that look like flower parts or butterfly wings hold your precious insides . . . well, inside. The two *pubococcygeus* muscles stretch from the pubic bone in front to the tailbone (coccyx) in back, like a mirror image, one on each side of the central urethra, the vaginal opening, and anus. Another pair are the *coccygeus* muscles, which connect the tailbone in back to the bones at the right and left sides of the pelvic basin. External pelvic muscles and structures reinforce both pairs. The perineum, which lies between your vaginal opening and the anus, is like a band that stretches from this center out to the right and left, connecting to the sides of the pelvic basin like an arched rainbow.

The pelvic floor also contains two sphincters. A sphincter is like a donut of muscle: if you clench it, you can stop things from passing in or out. We have one muscle sphincter around the urethra and vagina and another around the anus. To feel which muscles these are, try an experiment. Sit on the toilet when you are passing a stream of urine. Tighten the muscles to stop the stream of urine. Let it go. Stop it again. Release. You have just done two pelvic floor exercises!

Now that you know from the experiment which muscles to "feel," repeat this tightening and letting go when you are not passing urine. Repeat and count muscle contractions in groups of ten, fifteen groups of four, or whatever numbers you like and feel best doing. Hold for longer or increase the number of repetitions at your own pace. You can do these for any reason and at any time: standing at the sink making dinner, during intercourse, sitting in your car at a stoplight, standing in line, chatting on the phone. Not only will these exercises improve muscle tone when repeated frequently, but they also can improve orgasms and help the recovery of vaginal tone after delivery.

Nourishing Herbal Salve for Vaginal Comfort

Fill a clean, dry, wide-mouthed glass pint jar with 3 ounces of dried herb: 2 ounces wild yam, 1 ounce St. John's wort. Pour in 6 to 7 ounces of your choice of oil—for example, green, unfiltered, unheated olive oil, barely scented sweet almond oil, or safflower oil. Use enough oil to completely cover the herbs. You should be able to barely stir to the bottom of the jar with a table knife or wooden chopstick. To prevent contamination, wipe the edges of the jar clean and dry before fitting on a tight lid. Leave in a warm location for ten days—either keep on "low" in a slow cooker away from the reach of small children, or place the jar in a pot half full of warm water and set it in an oven heated only by the pilot light, or on a sunny windowsill, or on top of a water heater. The usual precaution about keeping herbal preparations away from heat and light doesn't apply here; in fact, it is the low heat that draws the herbal properties into the oil, but without getting the oil hot enough to turn it rancid.

After ten days or so, filter out the oil from the herb in muslin or cheesecloth. It will take a little hand-wringing over a colander or bowl, so wear an apron. Discard the oily herb (use as compost; roses especially love herb oils). Put the strained herb oil into an enamel or a stainless-steel saucepan over the lowest heat possible. Melt in equal amounts of coconut oil and cocoa butter—for example, 1 ounce strained herb oil, 1 ounce coconut oil, 1 ounce cocoa butter. As an option, you may want to add beeswax to add stability and thickness to your salve: use ⅛ ounce (about the size of a walnut) for every ounce of oil.

To predict the consistency your salve will have when it has cooled and solidified, dip a metal spoon into the oily mixture while it is warm. Put the spoon on a small plate in the refrigerator for five to ten minutes. After checking how the cooled mixture feels, add more of what's needed according to your preference: oil makes it more liquid, cocoa butter makes it soft but solid at room temperature, and beeswax makes it the most solid. Retest the consistency by refrigerating a dipped spoon as necessary. It may take sixty to ninety minutes for a larger amount (4 to 6 ounces) to cool down and solidify completely at room temperature.

Water and oil don't mix, especially in this recipe, so be careful not to get any water into the mixture. When you are satisfied with its consistency, pour the liquid salve into a clean jar with a tight-fitting lid.

Note: The rubber seals on canning jars go goopy after a while. Plain plastic or metal lids that fit well are better.

Congratulations—you have made an herbal salve! Use a teaspoon at a time for daily moisturizing or whenever lubrication makes more love happen. You may want to experiment with other combinations after trying the basic recipe a couple of times. Find more products like this in the Resources section.

Balancing complex health concerns through natural therapy is similarly incremental. The goal is to reestablish hormonal balance by correcting each hormonal center gradually, not by treating each separate symptom in turn. This is not a concept accepted by conventional Western medicine; this is Western *herbal* medicine. The hormonal tonic herbs help the liver, digestion, circulation, or nerves as well as support balanced endocrine function. This slow but sure process avoids many of the side effects caused when herbs are taken in large doses to combat symptoms, allowing each woman's own body to regulate itself and establish its natural hormonal balance as soon as possible. No matter what seems a little "off balance," you can safely take the combinations given as tea blends or combined tinctures during premenopause to balance the entire wheel of self-regulation.

Perimenopause may take you by surprise. Sometimes it catches us unaware and unprepared because we are focused on other health issues or life challenges during the years preceding middle age. But for us today, embracing all the changes of menopause can be, as it is in many cultures, the beginning of true wisdom. Achieving wisdom does not mean acting old; it means acting with the power that knowledge and experience bring. Now, even as we venture into a new millennium, more women are reaching back to prehistory for the tools that optimum health requires today. Herbal remedies to strengthen us along our journey are one way to open doors; what lies beyond we have only dreamed of. But knowledge of ancient and modern tools is not enough. We can know something full well yet not act on our knowledge. To be empowered demands action, even if it is simply the internal steps we take inside ourselves. Only when we take action to ensure our own well-being are we free to respond to the unpredictable challenges of this hormonal rite of initiation.

chapter 2
Menopause

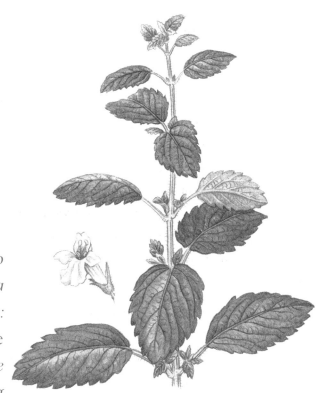

The word menopause–a combination of two Greek words, men and pausis–literally means a pause in menses. This life stage is unique to humans: no other animals go through it. Also known as the change of life or simply the Change, menopause occurs when our ovaries have stopped releasing the eggs they contained at birth. A strict definition of menopause is a complete cessation of menstrual periods. One year after your last menstrual flow you are postmenopausal. In common usage, however, it refers to the whole extent of time in which a woman's cycle is changing (the more formal term is perimenopause, and it is also called the climacteric).

Natural menopause may begin any time from age thirty-six to sixty; in the vast majority of women, it begins at about fifty-one. The biomedical view is that forty-five to fifty-five is the decade when natural menopause is most common; earlier than forty-five, doctors look for problems: history of cigarette smoking, primary ovarian failure, illness. However, in other cultures, mid-thirties perimenopause is not interpreted as illness. After nineteen years in practice among the affluent and underpriveleged, I noticed that mid-thirties women who took care of themselves did occasionally present with what seemed to be natural menopause without disease. But it is the extreme young edge of the range by any measure. Unless you get a blood test for elevated FSH (follicle-stimulating hormone) and LH, which most women don't bother with unless they are having severe symptoms, only in hindsight can you be diagnosed as having gone through menopause. The average length of the menopausal transition is just over a year, but it can last for several years. After twelve months without menstrual bleeding or pregnancy, a woman is considered to be "done" with menopause. But even this is not an absolute: some women are surprised by an erratic return of the menstrual cycle when they change their diets, fall in love, or start taking herbs. Some women joke that the word *menopause* means there are "many pauses" in their blood flow before it is over.

Menopause is signaled by some common signs and symptoms, but women experience them in varying intensity. According to various statistics, approximately 80 percent of women in the United States go through menopause with minimal discomfort but noticeable symptoms, including hot flashes and night sweats. For 10 percent of women it is a barely noticeable transition in terms of uncomfortable symptoms, and for the remaining 10 percent, there may be considerable discomfort associated with their menopausal transition. At menopause, other health problems that have been beneath the surface may worsen. For example, circulatory problems, cardiovascular problems, and rheumatic problems such as arthritis may become more troublesome.

Keep a simple diary for yourself and your health-care provider to assist you in describing your body's changes. Note the following:

* Cycle dates
* Length of periods
* Number of tampons, pads used
* Breast tenderness
* Mucus secretions or changes
* Hot flashes
* Disturbed nights of sleep
* Stress
* Exercise, which by itself has been shown to reduce all of the troubling symptoms in the list, to some degree!

As women enter this new stage of life, experiencing menopause's physiological changes, they also may identify new emotional and spiritual challenges in their lives and reevaluate their previous ways of living and their cultural beliefs. Menopause is unsettling enough in and of itself, but it also requires us to fend off negative social beliefs about what it is to be a woman and what it means, challenging us to confront Western society's perceptions about aging and older women and our preoccupation with youth, and to accept this new stage of life as a natural transformation. In cultures with a greater respect for elders, menopause is considered more as a natural rite of passage and less as a problem.

Added to all these concerns is the notion—held by ourselves and others—that anything that is natural, including menopause, should be a snap. We're all familiar with this myth: somewhere out in the world are women who always eat right, always stay in emotional equilibrium, and sail through menopause without complications or need for medication. This is the easiest notion about menopause to dispel. Though some women have no problems, if you do have difficulty, that does not mean you are somehow inadequate or blameworthy. Certainly we can be more forgiving to ourselves than that.

On the deepest level, women in menopause can find their new prime, though to do so they must release their old selves, and they must then discover anew who they are. There is an awareness of the mortality of one's physical body, which can be a liberating or a frightening revelation depending on a woman's belief system. It is not surprising that most women have some feelings of depression or uncertainty during these years. We may ponder the meaning of our lives thus far or feel overwhelmed by the possible paths still ahead of us before our ultimate physical passing. Thoughts of death are natural; contemplation of suicide is something far more serious. Pondering the passage of form is different than feeling like killing oneself. Hormonal swings and hitting emotional deep seas are not a sign you need biochemical balancing with antidepressants or other treatments. If this seems confusing, let's be clear: Suicidal thoughts are beyond a fleeting "I just want to die." If you think about ending it, see a licensed professional. Call a hotline. Ask for help. If, instead, your feelings bounce around, let's acknowledge that erratic emotions and feeling "crazy" are all part of menopause. Also, taking stock of one's life can raise feelings of regret, rage, and frustration. These are all important to accept, and when possible, to take steps toward transformation. That is a fine outcome to all those sweaty nights of sleep deprivation. This is a great time for some counseling or a life coach. Sharing experiences and feelings with good friends or seeking professional counseling may free you from your private fears as you go through this challenging transition. As you face the challenge of menopause, it's important to keep it in perspective: menopause is not a disease requiring treatment; it is a natural biological change.

Above all, we need to realize that after a temporary period of trial, whether mild or intense, every woman can enter the second half of her life with a wisdom and dignity no maiden can match.

Given all the challenges presented by menopause, a woman's choices to help with this transition range from the most simple remedies (such as rest and mild herbs) to the more complex, including hormone replacement therapy and surgery. To choose well, a woman of power simply needs to understand all her options.

The rest of this chapter explores common menopausal health conditions and the use of herbs to encourage a positive menopausal transformation. For centuries, simple and safe plant remedies have made the outward signs of this internal change more agreeable. In addition, general tips on whole-food nutrition for all the specific conditions discussed in this chapter can be found in the following "Herbs and Nutrition in Menopause" section.

herbs and nutrition in menopause

Being too thin doesn't give our bodies the the extra fat that helps cushion the decrease in estrogen, because fat cells make estrogen—our main supply once the ovaries stop doing this job. Being overweight, however, is not beneficial because after menopause our heart disease and diabetes risks go up.

We can define ideal weight, but did you know studies show that half of men surveyed and 85 percent of women are unhappy with their weight? Checkout stands and media outlets show us repeated visions of anorexic fifteen-year-olds to sell just about everything. We don't all meet the image presented, nor should we. Let's focus on healthy weight after getting the "ideal" put into perspective.

This is a time to love our bodies and both embrace our natural, unique, beautiful shapes and think about body weight in terms of health. Fad diets, obsessive aerobics, and starvation are antagonistic to the vibrancy that can be yours when you relax into the Change. A healthy weight and a steady routine of physical activity should be the goal. Women *can* control their weight and appearance, without going to extremes, as they change during menopause.

The wild card determining your ease or difficulty with this rite of passage may hinge on your attitude. Eating wisely may break a few calorie-counting rules and requires you to keep an open mind. Your body does not look as it did when you were sixteen, nor should it: you are a fully mature woman. Try seeing yourself with loving, not critical eyes, letting out the hidden feminine power within.

A varied, unrefined whole-food diet based on grains, fresh fruits, and vegetables in season may help ease the transition. Especially nourishing are wheat germ (for vitamin E), yogurt (soy or dairy—for low-fat energy, calcium, and strong intestinal flora), apricots (for iron), garlic (to lesson our risk of heart disease), and sprouted seeds and beans such as alfalfa, mung, and even onions (for essential fatty acids to protect nerves, quick energy, and some safe, food-based estrogen). Women who have an easier menopause tend to avoid excess protein and phosphorous-rich foods, red meat, refined flour, sugar and junk food, additives, added salt, smoking, alcohol, and caffeine (including chocolate and many brands of diet sodas). A temporary break from hot spices is also helpful.

continued on page 38

Foods rich in plant estrogens, or phytoestrogens (mild vegetable hormones with effects similar to those of natural estrogen in humans), are highly recommended during menopause. In a British study, twenty-three menopausal women ate foods rich in phytoestrogens—soy flour, red clover sprouts, and flaxseeds in an amount equal to 10 percent of their daily calories—for two weeks. During that time period, the degree of vaginal cell maturation (a sign of estrogen levels) went up significantly, causing the researchers to theorize that estrogen pills would be obsolete if women ate these foods. These findings were corroborated by an Australian study in which women averaging fifty-nine years ate 45 grams (1½ ounces) of soy flour every day for two weeks, then 25 grams (about 1 ounce) of linseed (flaxseed) meal daily for two weeks, then 10 grams (⅓ ounce) of red clover sprouts daily for two weeks. Again, vaginal cell maturation showed significant improvement that lasted another two weeks after the women stopped using these foods.

Eating well most of the time is a strong way of stabilizing your body's ever-changing neurochemical soup. The following lists are not absolute, but they do provide guidelines about foods to avoid and foods to increase in your regular eating patterns.

THE "LOW" TO "NO" CONSUMPTION LIST

* Fats, especially animal fats such as cheese and red meat. Aim to eat less than 30 to 40 grams of fat a day, or less than 10 to 30 percent of your daily calories in fat.

* Excess protein, beyond 10 to 20 percent of your daily caloric intake, or 50 grams, whichever is easier to track

* Packaged convenience foods

* Refined flour, sugar, junk food

* Additives (especially monosodium glutamate [MSG])

* Table salt, including excess "natural" sodium in tamari, soy sauce, and similar items

* Alcohol (especially red wine). First, red wine aggravates hot flashes and night sweats even more than other forms of alcohol do. Despite the many antioxidant benefits of resveratrol in red wine, alcohol consumption by women is known to be a risk factor for breast cancer. To get all the benefits of resveratrol without the alcohol, sensitive women can drink pomegranate juice or organic grape juice, avoiding the cancer-causing chemicals in commercial crops.

  Postmenopausally, fresh vegetable and carrot juices taken daily reduce risk of dementia, as does moderate alcohol consumption.

* Caffeine (including chocolate and sodas, diet sodas)

* Nicotine

* In addition, avoid overdependence on phosphorous-rich foods, such as a mono-diet of legumes, yellow corn, nuts, and parsnips—because phosphorous and calcium compete for the honor of being in your body. Eating too much phosphorous in an unbalanced diet diminishes calcium. However, the phytosterols of many legumes (peas, beans) and the essential fatty acids of raw nuts and seeds (almonds, sesame) have tremendous benefits for menopausal women. As with most things in life, the key here is moderation and common sense.

THE "YES" CONSUMPTION LIST

* Whole grains (brown rice, buckwheat, whole wheat with bran and wheat germ, whole oats, other grains)

* Fresh fruit in season, organic if possible

- Red, yellow, and green vegetables

- Various root vegetables (carrots, beets, burdock in soup, turnips, rutabaga, raw jicama in salads)

- Leafy green vegetables, organic if possible—all kinds

- Food sources of iron. Naturally occurring iron is more easily assimilated and will not cause constipation, unlike many iron supplements. Good choices include unsulfured dried apricots, soaked a few hours in springwater (making them easier to digest); raw pumpkin seeds (½ tablespoon sprinkled on salads); and blackstrap molasses. If you are not used to the taste of molasses, try a little, which tastes better than a lot at once. A very healthful breakfast is old-fashioned oatmeal porridge or another hot cereal served with a teaspoon of molasses and a few golden or brown raisins, to taste. Instant or microwaved starch-in-five-minutes-style oatmeal is not a brilliant example of Western civilization's progress; give it a pass. You can make real oatmeal almost as quickly: organic rolled oats take only five to fifteen minutes to cook once the water is boiling.

- Sprouted seeds and legumes. For good-quality essential fatty acids (helpful to immunity, nerves, and hormonal balance), enzymes (for overall metabolism and especially good digestion of proteins), and easily digested protein, make liberal use of these nutritional powerhouses. You can find sprouts at natural-food stores or you can purchase dried seeds and sprout them at home. Soy, sunflower, aduki, fenugreek, onion, and other live green sprouts provide an array of vitamins, minerals, phytoestrogens, and chlorophyll to sweeten the belly and the breath.

- Diuretic foods that help prevent water retention and bloating: these include freshly grated cabbage, cucumber, pineapple, parsley, watermelon, and cantaloupe. Cabbage, broccoli, and brussels sprouts have health benefits, including cancer prevention, but eaten in excess they may worsen digestive gas, so use them to the extent you find best for your needs. Vitamin B_6, also a diuretic, is needed even more than usual by women who have taken the Pill, because after three years of use the Pill decreases assimilation of B_6. Low B_6 is also associated with diabetes, and good blood sugar stability is associated with the whole B vitamin complex.

- The B vitamin complex (found in whole grains, legumes, dairy, animal products), which not only stabilizes blood sugar but also ensures healthy nerves. You can get enough from nonanimal sources with a balanced whole-food diet.

- When optimizing liver function is important—as with hepatitis, a past history of substance abuse, or other liver damage—add the herb milk thistle (*Silybum marianus*) to the diet (1 tablespoon of seeds daily). These nutty-tasting, rice-size brown seeds can be freshly ground in a coffee grinder and added to foods such as salad dressings, protein drinks, fruit smoothies, and soups, or sprinkled over cooked grains. Milk thistle helps protect regenerating liver cells. Larger amounts can be taken as a supplement if needed.

- A word about the tendency to overuse multivitamins and supplements: in general, don't rely on tablets for your basic nutrition; they are hard to digest and may not be assimilated well. Worse, in my opinion, overuse of particular supplements may condition the body to slack off on some of its functions; sometimes the body will perform certain digestive processes only if you chew those enzyme supplements you've been taking regularly with your food. Try choosing foods that you enjoy and that supply the basic nutrition you need, and leave the supplements for only those genuine deficiencies that satisfying nutritional foods cannot resolve.

CARDIOVASCULAR DISEASE

In recent years, estrogen's protection against diseases of the cardiovascular system (CVS) has been big news, with the risk of cardiovascular disease said to be related to a woman's level of estrogen. Though this is not the whole story, conventional medicine and popular media have repeatedly told women that after menopause we catch up with men in terms of heart attacks, strokes, and other heart disease. Statistics suggest this is true. Yet beyond numbers, lifestyle and aging have more to do with heart health in men and women than missing or replacing hormones. Now new studies are questioning the cardiovascular benefits of hormone replacement therapy and estrogen replacement therapy (discussed more fully in chapter 3).

With or without hormones complicating the scene, medical researchers have not yet uncovered all the facts about heart disease. Yes, serum cholesterol and triglycerides (blood fats) do go up after the Change. The drop in estrogen around this age is assumed to be the single major cause, and higher blood fat levels and low estrogen do occur together. But these two body changes by themselves do not lead to myocardial infarctions (heart attacks), especially if a woman was not at risk for a heart attack anyway (see "Risk Factors for Cardiovascular Disease" on page 41). Furthermore, the medical model of reducing cholesterol and LDLs (low-density lipoproteins or "bad," cholesterol-laden fats) misses the point about improving heart health. Because estrogen has been studied as an isolated hormone, its effects may have been taken out of context. The body has complex ways of staying in balance. In menopause a woman's body reacts to changes in estrogen levels, yet menopause is more than a single effect of any one chemical, even chemicals as potent as hormones. We do know that estrogen affects the cardiovascular system by increasing heart-protecting HDLs (high-density lipoproteins or "good" fats) that counteract LDLs. Meanwhile, estrogen stimulates more than four hundred types of cells that have estrogen receptors, so giving it as a replacement in menopause affects more than the heart and blood.

Progesterone's role in postmenopausal heart disease is also unclear. Blamed for lowering HDL, progesterone can also help us by lowering blood fats. Women still have some progesterone throughout the Change, so in the past, conventional medical researchers assumed that to lower the menopause-related risks of heart disease, women needed to be dosed with estrogen. But today fewer women are taking estrogen by itself because it carries with it an increased risk of cancers (uterine lining, endometrial, and perhaps others). The conventional medical opinion is that if a woman no longer has her uterus, it is okay to prescribe estrogen alone for preventing CVS risks, but estrogen does increase risks of other health concerns, including breast cancer. The combination of estrogen and progesterone (HRT), which is considered safer, is commonly prescribed to women who have not had a hysterectomy. Nevertheless, studies do not agree that HRT gives the same cardiovascular

risk factors for cardiovascular disease

High-fat diet	High blood pressure
High salt intake	Emotional or physical stress or trauma
Smoking	Obesity
Diabetes	High cholesterol, especially high LDLs
Family history	and low HDL
Lack of exercise	

benefits as estrogen alone. The picture remains confused. One study of women of the same age, some premenopausal and others in menopause, showed they had different estrogen levels but the same cardiovascular risks. It appears that the presence or absence of estrogen in menopause is not the biggest cause of women's higher heart attack rates after menopause. On a positive note, conventional science has debunked the myth of cardiovascular protection from HRT, so fewer doctors recommend it, though it is still found on some contemporary websites giving medical advice to menopausal women.

In reality, postmenopausal heart disease may have more to do with unhealthy lifestyles than the lack of estrogen. Indeed, postmenopausal heart attacks have been on the rise since World War II, a period in which more women have been smoking, eating fast foods high in fats and salt, and working at full-time jobs outside the home. Heart problems in older women today are more likely due to weight, the ratio of HDL (good) to LDL (bad) fats, family history of heart problems, smoking, lifelong health, or recent patterns of nutrition and exercise. Add to this the effects of stress on the heart, and we can see that the problem of heart disease should not be explained away as a menopausal "lack" of estrogen.

Medicine already supports this idea, because it is well known that, for example, by making commonsense changes in our diets and not smoking we can lower cardiovascular risks. Natural therapists suggest that in addition to adopting healthy habits, you may be able to lower heart attack risks another way: by making midlife the time for opening your heart to what is, rather than pining for what is past. This change of life for both men and women requires a "change of heart"—new ways of coping with life's challenges for fulfillment at this age. We know a go-getter attitude or a stressful style of approaching life's ups and downs is part of the makeup of those most likely to suffer heart disease. A healing response to heart problems may be to change stressful work patterns, old patterns of eating and carousing, and feelings of hard-heartedness in an emotional relationship.

Some research suggests that menopausal symptoms are better balanced by giving progesterone rather than adding estrogen. This may explain why herbs found to be helpful for menopause do not all necessarily have estrogenic effects. Several traditional remedies for hot flashes and other menopausal symptoms instead promote the body's production of progesterone and related hormones.

A last note about heart health, fat, and hormones: when women in the Change are in anything resembling reasonable health, androgens (masculine sex hormones) are still present as part of the hormonal mix. These are gradually changed into estrone (a type of estrogen) in the adrenal glands, in fat cells, and elsewhere. For this reason, maintaining a healthy, protective number of fat cells will naturally provide more estrone, which in turn means fewer problems from the loss of estrogen produced by the ovaries—a good argument for keeping a little cushion of body fat while maintaining fitness—and a good argument against the obsessively excessive attention some women place on reducing to a fat-free, bone-thin, androgynous body type.

Herbal Medicine

The following herbal formulas help the entire cardiovascular system, especially for those women who are in higher-risk groups. Although the herbs also help with hot flashes, they are specifically designed to strengthen blood vessels and heart muscle, normalize blood pressure, and improve circulation to the fingers and toes. They will not cause negative interactions with medication for high blood pressure and are safe for children and men to drink, too.

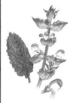
Concentrate for cardiovascular support

CONCENTRATED HERB EXTRACT	ACTIONS
4 oz. hawthorn leaf, flower, berry (*Crataegus species*)	Safely relaxes blood vessels; lowers high blood pressure
1 oz. motherwort herb (*Leonurus cardiaca*)	Lessens hot flashes; calms a pounding heart
1½ tsp. blackstrap molasses	Nutritive; provides iron without causing constipation
2 fluid oz. plus 1½ tbsp. black cherry juice concentrate (available at natural-food stores)	For taste; to harmonize strong herbal actions

Combine all ingredients. Take 1 teaspoon once or twice a day, diluted in 1 cup of water, juice, or any herb tea, in the morning and evening.

Eight ounces will last two to three weeks.

Tea for cardiovascular support

DRIED HERBS	ACTIONS
2 oz. linden flower (*Tilia* species*)*	Moistens; relaxes; tones blood vessels and nerves
2 oz. hawthorn flower, leaf (*Crataegus* species*)*	Nourishes heart; stabilizes circulation
2 oz. hawthorn berry (*Crataegus* species*)*	Nourishes heart; stabilizes circulation
½ oz. hibiscus flower (*Hibiscus sabdariffa*)	For taste; cooling; nutritive
1½ oz. lemon balm leaf (*Melissa officinalis*)	Soothes digestion; for taste

Put ½ ounce of the mixture and 3 cups of boiling water in a teapot or container with a well-fitting lid. Let stand for fifteen minutes before straining. Drink 1 cup, hot or cold, one to three times a day.

Eight ounces will last approximately two weeks at 3 cups a day, up to forty-eight days at 1 cup a day.

Nutrition

Review the following suggestions for whole foods that provide vitamins and minerals to address cardiovascular health, along with the list of natural supplements.

wise food choices

❀ Eat smaller meals more often.

❀ Limit fats in the diet to 10 to 20 percent of total daily calories (not the 30 percent allowed by conventional dietitians or the 45 percent common in the American diet).

❀ If you choose to eat eggs, use them in moderation. Even in a low-fat diet, two or three non-fried eggs per week are fine. No matter how many commercials by egg and dairy lobbies you see, choose organic and free-range eggs. (Nonorganic eggs are loaded with hormones and chemicals. Free-range chickens that scratch around in organic soil for minerals, bugs, and grains produce healthier eggs and a healthier environment than miserably caged hens fed antibiotics under commercial production conditions.)

❀ Increase intake of vitamin E for its antioxidant benefits and its role in helping older people cope with stress and aging. It occurs naturally in vegetable oils, eggs, unprocessed cereals, some fish and meat, and leafy vegetables. Sprouted seeds, besides being rich in essential fatty acids that nourish the skin and the immune system, provide vitamin E, enzymes, and readily digestible protein. Avocados, wheat germ, and flaxseed are other food sources of vitamin E.

❀ Use healthy fats (HDLs) to help prevent cardiovascular disease. Omega-3 fatty acids are found in seafood; other helpful fatty acids are found in oats and dried beans (legumes), so enjoy oatmeal and split pea soup!

❀ One clove of raw or lightly steamed garlic a day is preventative for high cholesterol, hardened arteries, and other factors of heart disease. Women in higher-risk groups can eat more, up to three cloves a day. Try taking a raw clove, finely chopped and mixed well with a few tablespoons of applesauce. It is easy to swallow, especially if you're quick. Or press one clove into 1 teaspoon of honey and knock it back with water. It goes down easily without causing a headache or stomach upset—but not on an empty stomach. Even if you love garlic, you'll know you are at the upper limit of what your body can use if you start to get an upset stomach, in which case take a break from it or try less. If you can't take much garlic, try these alternatives: Add it finely chopped to steamed vegetables, soups, or rice during the last five to ten minutes of cooking. Add a handful of finely chopped parsley or a teaspoon of dried leaves, freshly crumbled between your palms, to the dish before eating. After dinner, sweeten your breath by nibbling on a few cardamom seeds. If you just can't eat garlic, deodorized capsules and tablets are available; take as directed on the label. If these don't agree with you, don't worry about missing the benefits of garlic—it isn't the only way to help your heart.

❀ Increase fiber in the form of vegetables, fruit, and whole grains (for example, whole oats have more nutritional value and are cheaper than oat bran).

❀ Limit intake of caffeine, as it raises blood pressure, blood fats, and your risk of heart disease.

❀ Limit alcohol use; one glass of wine or beer with the evening meal may help some people lower their risk of heart disease, but for most people larger amounts over time increase the risk of cardiovascular disease and many other illnesses.

❀ Avoid animal fats from red meat, chicken, cheese, milk, and rich seafood. However, seafood is rich in omega-3 fatty acids, which are helpful in preventing heart disease. If you choose to eat seafood, emphasize white or lean fish, which are lower in calories than lobster, crab, salmon, and sardines, all of which are high in fat. Fatty seafood is great for getting omega-3s; just don't eat it every day as a preventative therapy!

❀ Avoid hydrogenated or partially hydrogenated fats (margarine, many packaged foods, snack items).

❀ Avoid salt and monosodium glutamate (MSG). We get more than enough sodium in vegetables, grains, proteins, and whole foods. An excess of added table salt leads to water retention, high blood pressure, and other complaints.

supplements

❀ If you have problems enjoying garlic, try deodorized capsules; take as directed on product labels.

* To quickly lower cholesterol, try fiber, especially psyllium, flax, or chia seeds. Mix 1 teaspoon powdered seeds in an 8-ounce glass of water (if soaked for any length of time, the seeds will form a gelatinous mixture). Or take them in capsules as directed on product labels, making sure to drink eight glasses of water during the day. If you do not drink this extra water, the fiber will absorb much of your body's water, possibly creating some constipation. This is why cooked grains, legumes, or fresh whole vegetables, which contain the right amount of water for their fiber content, are better than fiber supplements in the long term.

* Omega-3 fatty acids are anti-inflammatory, decrease the risk of strokes, and lower blood fats. Several products are available; use as directed on labels.

In Addition

* Exercise according to your body type and favorite movements.

* Stop smoking. It is never too late, and it will do you a world of good.

* Meditate (see "Opening the Heart Meditation" on page 46).

OSTEOPOROSIS

Osteoporosis, the depletion of calcium in our bones, is a big concern for women throughout menopause. Bones affected by this disease are porous and weakened, which may lead to fractures, back pain, loss of height, and stooped posture. The condition is quite common and increases with age; according to the National Institutes of Health, osteoporosis is a major public health threat for forty-four million Americans—68 percent of whom are women—and half of all U.S. women over fifty will experience an osteoporosis-related fracture in their lifetime (see www.niams.nih.gov/Health_Info/Bone/Osteoporosis/default.asp).

As women go through menopause, the drop in estrogen affects the bones' ability to retain calcium. Until menopause, estrogen has a stimulating effect on our body's bone-building activity throughout life. Around puberty, sudden increases of estrogen provide extra stimulation for growth spurts. Later, through our reproductive years, estrogen stimulates the continued formation of strong bones to pick up our growing children or to handle the mineral loss of menstruation. After our reproductive years, the decreased stimulation of bones by estrogen can be compensated for by continuing exercise and optimizing bone strength with all the factors in our control. Those that natural therapies can address follow in these pages.

You may not realize you are developing osteoporosis because it occurs gradually at the cellular level. We all have two types of bone cells. The osteoblasts (bone makers) are cells that take minerals from the bloodstream and use them to build concentric rings of strong bone. Their opposite twin

Opening the Heart Meditation

If you record this meditation, you may wish to leave a silent pause of thirty seconds or more where asterisks (*) appear. Find five minutes in a quiet spot and sit or lie in a comfortable position. Close your eyes for the meditation.

Count your breath evenly and slowly. * Now tune in to the beating of your heart. It is a drumbeat. Let it sound evenly and slowly with your breath. No other thoughts or feelings are allowed to interrupt your loving attention to your natural rhythmic heartbeat. In your mind's eye, you see or imagine that your heart is not only red, but also green, like a garden. It is cool and moist, very tender. Some places in the garden of your heart are hot and strong, like a magnificent crimson rose, a passionate river of lava, capable of changing the world.

As you slowly stroll through your garden, you stop and admire the beauty and fragrance of the flowers bending over the path. At your feet are a few weeds sprouting here and there. You talk to them, saying you will change their physical form now. You find yourself easily uprooting the ones you can see. You recognize these weeds in your imaginary garden of the heart as the hard words spoken yesterday or an old envy, a missed joy. As you remove the weeds from the path winding through your inner landscape of emotions, name them if you can. When you have weeded enough for today, visualize yourself carrying the limp remains of the plants out of the garden, and place them where they may decompose into rich earth for tomorrow's flowers.

As you face your garden before leaving, you notice that the flowers have doubled since you last looked. Your dark thoughts have been freed. Sun and shadow dance in your heart.

Tune in to the beat of your heart once more. Count your breathing slowly and evenly. * When you feel ready, bring your full attention back to the place where you sit in silence.

Tending to this inner vision of your changing heart makes room for love, for both others and ourselves. In contemplation or in the physical realm, there is nothing like a little gardening, just five minutes here and there, to open your heart.

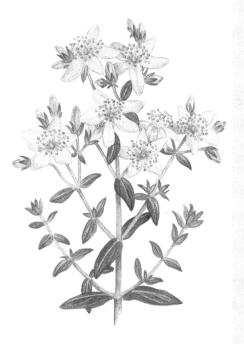

cells, the osteoclasts (bone *un*makers), are constantly taking away dense bone material and breaking it down to return minerals to the bloodstream. This natural and healthy process allows the bones to handle the body's constantly changing demand for minerals. We need calcium, vitamin D, and a variety of minerals in the blood for activities happening at the cellular level throughout the body. These activities include maintaining a steady heartbeat, keeping the kidneys' excretion of wastes in happy balance, and soothing our frazzled nerves. This exchange of minerals from bone to blood and from blood to bone ensures the bones are always in the process of being re-formed with new building materials.

Your level of physical activity provides stimulus for the osteoblasts, so that you make bones just as dense as your activity level demands. With movement, bones thicken the more they are used for a particular activity. This is the bones' natural response to body signals that they prepare for more of the same activity. Without regular body movement, bones have no good reason to be strong. Inactivity, not a decline in estrogen, is your bones' enemy. While you sit reading this book, your bones have dissolved a little of their calcium strength into the bloodstream, for whatever purpose the body needs.

In fact, weight-bearing exercise is widely seen as a major way to prevent osteoporosis. It's never too late to start, and even after menopause, weight-bearing exercise has been recently shown to significantly ameliorate osteoporosis, but the best effects are seen in women who begin regular moderate exercise at least by age thirty-five and continue beyond menopause.

Your exercise program should fit the level of your tolerance or fitness, and it should be a pleasurable discipline that can be done often. Anything that combines muscle contraction and the good effects of gravity's pull on your bones will help prevent bone loss, so good choices are walking, running, dancing, uphill walking, and weight training. At the very least, keep your posture straight and walk a lot. While swimming is not weight-bearing, pushing against the resistance of the water is an excellent start for women with weak joints or weight problems. To make it fun, seek out support groups or friends with whom you actually enjoy exercising.

Like exercise, estrogen stimulates the osteoblasts to turn calcium in the bloodstream into dense bone. This is why estrogen replacement has historically been presented to women as a treatment or prevention for osteoporosis. Not all women with osteoporosis break their hips, and not all middle-aged or elderly women with fractures have a bone density problem. Some women with hip fractures have bone densities similar to those who don't break any bones. In general, osteoporosis studies do not consider other possible causes of broken bones in women: the isolation of greater numbers of single aging women, poverty among the elderly, public safety, or housing conditions.

There is more to osteoporosis than the exercise and estrogen issues. Even without definitive proof about their efficacy, calcium supplements are widely recommended to middle-aged women for prevention of osteoporosis. Yet calcium is one of the most abundant, widely available minerals in whole foods, so we are not likely to be calcium deficient through diet. Do we automatically need to consume between 1 and 2 grams of calcium per day (an average dose of 1,200 to 1,500 milligrams), in addition to whatever is in our salad bowls? This high amount is still standard advice, whether from physicians, newspaper medical columnists, or some alternative health publications, whose advertisers make calcium or multimineral supplements. The challenge is to *absorb* the calcium and other minerals we are already eating in our diets.

Getting calcium from the food we eat is our best option. However, the sad truth at the time of this writing is that most older women do not and often cannot get adequate intake from their diets through greens. It can be hard enough for elder women to shop. Still, for most women, the calcium from many whole foods—called *bioavailable calcium*—is easily absorbed in the digestive process, which makes it bioavailable. Some examples of calcium-rich vegetables include slightly bitter greens such as kale and chard, which also encourage healthy stomach acid, necessary for calcium assimilation. Many commercial calcium supplements, on the other hand, have an alkaline carrier (antacids) that neutralizes stomach acids, making calcium absorption far less likely. Look for products that list sources of calcium other than calcium carbonate, such as calcium citrate or calcium malate. Taking larger amounts of supplements will not ensure better uptake. Besides, too much calcium carbonate can act like an alkaline chalk, interfering more seriously with acidic digestive juices. When these digestive secretions are the wrong pH, women can begin to have problems breaking down food, maintaining general immune resistance, and avoiding anemia. Another potential problem of excessive calcium supplementation is its effect on the kidneys, which clear the bloodstream when it is burdened with too much of this mineral. The kidneys excrete excess calcium via urine. Excess calcium can lead to urinary-tract problems, even kidney stones.

Calcium in the diet does not have to come from dairy products. In fact, nuts, seeds, and greens are more bioavailable sources of calcium and other nutrients for mature women than milk, cheese, antacids, or sugary colon cleansers. Taking vitamin D is another way women protect more than their bones, since this multipurpose supplement synergizes with calcium and several cofactors for total health as we age. The recommended dosage range is 400 to 800 milligrams per day. Vitamin D is discussed in more detail a little later. There are several other reasons to consume your leafy greens. Recent studies have shown the significance of vitamin K in preventing osteoporosis-related fractures. The level of vitamin K has been reported to be an indicator of bone mineral density as well as an indicator of potential hip fracture. It is produced by intestinal bacteria and can also be found in leafy green vegetables. Additionally, leafy greens (and all vegetables and fruits) are excellent sources of potassium. Increasing consumption of potassium-rich foods lowers urinary calcium excretion and decreases the risk of osteoporosis. Potassium also significantly reduces bone turnover. It is clear that leafy green vegetables should play a key role in the prevention of osteoporosis. This is partially because we need vitamins and minerals that are in natural proportions, as found in many whole foods. Leafy vegetables and other nondairy sources of calcium also help protect our hearts and may reduce our pain sensitivity; overdependence on animal products has the opposite effect. As animal protein is broken down in the digestive tract, the release of arachidonic acid leads to production of more inflammatory compounds called prostaglandins. These prostaglandins play a part in the development of joint pain and some chronic degenerative diseases considered "normal" in our culture as we age. Enjoying animal protein isn't the problem; overdependence is. Another concern with dairy products is the industry's use of antibiotic-laced cattle feeds and stimulating growth hormones.

Vegetable and nut sources of calcium are a greater part of diets in other parts of the world such as Asia, where women don't eat a lot of cheese, don't take calcium supplements, and don't have anything like our Western "epidemic" of osteoporosis. A clear correlation has been made between a culture's dairy consumption and the occurrence of osteoporosis, meaning that the more dairy products a society consumes in general, the more likely people are to develop osteoporosis. The Asian diet is traditionally lower than ours in meat and protein; dairy is rarely eaten. Asian women eat half or less of the calcium load that Western women consume, and their bones are not thinning nearly as rapidly as ours. They are also getting soy sources starting in pregnancy and other phytoestrogen rich foods from childhood, such as mung beans. For this reason, Asian women living traditionally have an overall estrogen decline that is different from women eating a standard North American diet. Further, they tend to incorporate a lot more weight-bearing exercise into their lifestyles. In Beijing, women do not drive to the supermarket, load packages of processed vegetable protein or even tofu into the back of the SUV, and drive home. They bicycle, walk, carry bags, and as a rule, tend to burn the phytoestrogen-rich fuel that is traditional in their diet. Asian cultures also consume more omega-3 fatty acids, the fats you get from fish, nuts, and seeds. A healthy amount of omega-3 fatty acids has been shown to minimize the decline in bone mass caused by menopause. You can achieve this amount by eating oily fish once a week, taking fish oil supplement, or making sure that a substantial amount of your dietary fats and oils come from healthy nuts and seeds, or olive oil. Ironically for women who believe they have to drink milk to strengthen their bones, the high protein in dairy products binds with dairy's calcium, making this mineral less available for the body's needs (bones, nerve impulses, healthy blood pH).

More recently, there has been a lot of information about vitamin D and osteoporosis. Vitamin D plays an important role in calcium absorption and in bone health. Most of the vitamin D in your body is created through exposure to sunlight, and although our bodies should be able to manufacture vitamin D from that exposure, many people who are elderly or who do not get enough sunlight exposure at northern latitudes are potentially deficient. Depending on your situation, you may need to take vitamin D supplements to ensure a daily intake of between 400 to 800 I.U. of vitamin D, although there is conflicting information about higher doses.

Other dietary risk factors for osteoporosis are a high-protein diet and high sodium intake. Eating a high-protein diet is one sure way to lose extra calcium and increase your risk for osteoporosis. Women who eat less salt, protein, and sugar than is common in the standard American diet (all of these rob calcium from the body) have less need, if any at all, for calcium supplements.

risk factors for osteoporosis

No exercise

Smoking

No pregnancies

Drinking alcoholic beverages daily (though moderate consumption is cardioprotective)

Caffeine and soda (more than a total of five cups a day)

Excess fat in diet, especially animal fats, including dairy products

High-protein diet

High-sodium diet

Calcium supplements, especially without magnesium (though a diet low in calcium is a risk factor, taking calcium in excess, as an isolated nutrient, is not as helpful and may even interfere with calcium bioavailability)

Being underweight by more than fifteen pounds

Being overweight by more than twenty-five pounds

Non-African-American ethnic group

Early onset of menstruation

Early menopause

Past medical history of pathological fracture (without obvious cause or trauma)

Family history of osteoporosis

Family history of diabetes

Steroid drugs, especially with long-term use because of arthritis, asthma, or autoimmune disorders

Thyroid medication, especially with long-term use

The National Women's Health Network has described, in addition, a social set of factors that do not show up on all the conventional lists of risks for older women and "pathological fracture" (breaking a bone without the usual force of trauma). In North America, pathological fracture happens most commonly to women over the age of seventy. Little-known cofactors include combined problems that are usually seen as unrelated, for instance, worsening eyesight and uneven curbs. Public safety is a concern as economic pressures cause local governments to postpone repairs. Poverty, or simply the malnutrition seen in older women who no longer prepare meals because they live alone, are other social factors associated with a rise in osteoporosis.

For women in the higher-risk group for osteoporosis (see page 50), prevention can begin years before menopause. Osteoporosis prevention begins in childhood! Women who begin a weight-bearing exercise program by age thirty-five can still reduce their risk. But if you have not yet taken precautions against bone thinning, it's still not too late. The truth is, for women who don't have a large number of risk factors, the best prevention is exercise, whole-food nutrition, and, when necessary, herbs to nourish the blood and bones and encourage healthy levels of post-menopausal hormones.

Please remember that it takes more than one risk factor to cause a multifactorial disease such as osteoporosis. Panic about having a few risk factors is not as helpful as changing what you can. When you have started to do that, you can relax about the few things you may not be able to change.

Herbal Medicine

In the following formulas, the diuretic action of dandelion leaf and root helps the kidneys excrete any excess calcium and avoid kidney stones, but never by removing it from bone. Dandelion leaf is also naturally rich in potassium, which we need when we take diuretics—yet another example of nature's inherent wisdom. This multipurpose herb is also a digestive bitter that helps rebalance normal stomach acid if you have been using an excess of calcium supplements.

Herbs rich in calcium and other minerals are best taken as a tea because the water assists in bio-availability. The next two combinations can also strengthen skin, nails, and hair in three or more months. If your mane becomes glossy and you run like the wind, just be careful when you start to sow those wild oats. If you have unstable high blood pressure or heart disease that is not well managed by prescriptions, there is a small possibility that excessive use (more than five cups of tea or five doses of tincture a day) may be too much of a good thing. See your health-care provider if you have questions or any worsening of health.

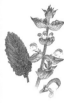

Concentrate for bone health

CONCENTRATED HERB EXTRACT	ACTIONS
2 oz. wild oat herb *(Avena sativa)*	Provides minerals; nourishes nerves, skin, hair
2 oz. horsetail herb *(Equisetum arvense)*	Helps kidneys, elimination; provides minerals
1 oz. dandelion root, raw *(Taraxacum officinale)*	Helps elimination, liver, digestion
1 oz. dandelion root, roasted *(Taraxacum officinale)*	Adds minerals; for taste
1 oz. dandelion leaf *(Taraxacum officinale)*	Reduces water retention; adds minerals
1 oz. nettle leaf *(Urtica dioica)*	Nutritive; supports immune resistance
1 oz. yellow dock root *(Rumex crispus)*	Stimulates liver; aids fat metabolism; adds iron
1 oz. alfalfa herb *(Medicago sativa)*	Nutritive; relieves stiffness; provides gentle hormonal effects

Combine these herbal extracts. Take 1 teaspoon twice a day (in the morning and evening) in 1 cup of water, juice, or any herb tea.

Ten ounces will last thirty days.

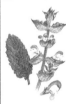

Tea for bone health

DRIED HERBS	ACTIONS
3 oz. wild oat herb *(Avena sativa)*	Provides minerals; nourishes nerves, skin, hair
2 oz. horsetail herb *(Equisetum arvense)*	Helps kidneys, elimination; provides minerals
2 oz. dandelion root, raw *(Taraxacum officinale)*	Helps elimination, liver, digestion
2 oz. dandelion root, roasted *(Taraxacum officinale)*	Adds minerals; for taste
2 oz. dandelion leaf *(Taraxacum officinale)*	Reduces water retention; adds minerals
2 oz. nettle leaf *(Urtica dioica)*	Nutritive; supports immune resistance
1 oz. yellow dock root *(Rumex crispus)*	Stimulates liver; aids fat metabolism; adds iron
1 oz. alfalfa herb *(Medicago sativa)*	Nutritive; relieves stiffness; provides gentle hormonal effects

Add ½ ounce of the mixture to 4 cups of boiling water in a teapot or container with a well-fitting lid. Let stand for twenty minutes before straining. Drink 1 cup, hot or cold, three times a day. Or if you prefer, sip tea all day or drink 2 large glasses twice a day—just be sure to drink 3 cups a day.

Fifteen ounces will last thirty days.

Nutrition

Review the following suggestions for whole foods that provide vitamins and minerals to address bone health, as well as the list of natural supplements.

wise food choices

❀ Calcium is widely available in nature, and most plants we eat have it in abundance, unless the only vegetables you eat are iceberg lettuce and commercially grown tomatoes. For non-dairy sources of calcium that are easy on your heart, cholesterol, and general health, and won't add pounds the way dairy foods can, eat dark green leafy vegetables, especially spinach, kale, dandelion greens, watercress, chard, and parsley. The leafy greens are also high in vitamin K and potassium, both important for strong bones. Fresh raw nuts and seeds such as almonds, sunflower seeds, pumpkin seeds, and particularly sesame seeds (including tahini) are also high in calcium and in omega-3 fatty acids.

❀ Vegetables can be steamed if the roughage causes digestive upsets. And do eat your spinach, even though it occasionally gets bad press. Yes, spinach contains oxalic acids that bind with calcium and decrease available iron, but it does different things when eaten raw, steamed, with other foods, or all by itself. Try preparing it as people in traditional Mediterranean cultures do: drizzle a little lemon juice or ½ teaspoon of raw organic apple cider vinegar over combinations of steamed or raw spinach and other green leafy vegetables; the acidic pH of the lemon juice makes the minerals in the greens more easily digestible. Though spinach has some oxalic acid, which should be avoided by people who are sensitive to its negative effects on arthritis, it is so full of chlorophyll and other good nutrients that people call it the "friend of the elderly."

❀ Each week eat at least two servings of beans and legumes, including tofu or tempeh—a high-protein soy food that is rich in calcium—instead of meat, fish, or eggs. Avoid brands with added preservatives. Fresh tofu and tempeh are available at natural-food stores or Asian groceries.

❀ Avoid refined sugars, which rob the body of calcium and interfere with blood sugar balance, energy, mood, and hormonal and immune system stability.

supplements

❀ If you choose to use calcium supplements, remember that natural vitamin D (not the synthetic one in milk) helps absorption. Also, women need to balance calcium the way nature does, with the right ratio of magnesium. If you truly need supplements, don't bother with ones containing an aluminum-based antacid or alkaline carrier, because they interfere with the stomach acid needed to absorb calcium. If you double your calcium, be sure to double your magnesium; it should always be half as much as your calcium intake. For example, if you take 1,200 milligrams of calcium, don't go by the RDA (recommended daily allowance) of 280 milligrams of magnesium for women; take 560 to 600 milligrams of magnesium.

* Get plenty of vitamin C, preferably from food sources, as described in "Hot Flashes and Night Sweats," page 67.

In Addition

* Exercise. In my experience, women hate it or love it. If you hate it, don't ever do it again. That's right. Because by *exercise*, I refer specifically to organized gym workouts or whatever you dislike or avoid. What you want to do is *move*. The general discussion on exercise earlier in this section provides suggestions on healthy ways to move. In most preindustrial and some contemporary cultures, physical exercise is not thought of "meeting a daily quota for exercise." It is simply movement, using one's body every day. Walking with groceries, gathering wood or water, or creating physical structures, whether art, garden, farm, or home, are examples of physical activities women incorporate into everyday life. Either way, in the gym or not, women who have physical activity do not seem to have to worry as much about osteoporosis, heart disease, and other risk factors for illness as we age.

* Now is the time to gain in physical fitness and drop excess weight—if at all possible, without self-judgment or getting depressed. Just start wherever you are.

* Avoid fluoride in toothpaste and water because it interferes with calcium absorption.

* Protect yourself from pollution—for example, by getting away to the country more often and by removing toxic chemicals from your home and yard.

* Check with your physician to see whether your medications (antacids with aluminum, heparin, steroids for arthritis, thyroid hormones, anticonvulsants) can be switched or reduced to minimize their effects on bone loss.

* Limit alcohol and caffeine to commonsense servings that provide antioxidant and other health benefits.

* Eliminate smoking.

DEPRESSION

The changes women undergo in the course of their lives have long seemed mysterious and were feared by men and women alike. Even at the turn of the twentieth century, some menopausal women were institutionalized for *involutional melancholia*, a term for menopausal depression. Conventional medicine continues to focus on pathology even where menopause is concerned, viewing the Change as a "failure" of the ovaries to produce adequate estrogen, and proposing surgical and pharmaceutical options to cure it. But menopausal women are not deficient. We are not failing. We may need supportive health advice but not automatic replacement of a hormone that the body was designed to lower at this time of life.

If you feel unable to cope with stress or your emotions seem out of control during menopause, the cause is likely to be changes in your hormonal balance, which is partly controlled by the adrenal glands. One job of the adrenal glands is to make adrenaline and other hormones that help us respond to stress. A related function is making small amounts of sex hormones. After menopause, the adrenal glands continue to make a little estrogen and other steroidal hormones, but mainly they take the androstenedione that our ovaries continue to produce and convert it into the hormone estrone, which has beneficial effects similar to those of estrogen. Therefore, taking care of your adrenals before and during menopause is a good way to ensure that you improve your changing tolerance to stress and depression. The herbs in the following formulas can help optimize adrenal health and also help you gain more natural control over your body's own balance of estrogen and its close relative, estrone.

After an initial period of unpredictability, you'll find that your response to stress improves as your body adjusts to its new hormonal balance. The process is similar to what happens after rearranging furniture: you are used to having it the old way, so initially you may bump into the furniture, but very soon you get used to the new pathways.

If you experience suicidal feelings during menopause, they are not necessarily a sign of severe mental disease, but rather of depression resulting from your changing hormonal balance. But by no means should you ignore these feelings: seek the company of a trusted friend or the counsel of a mental health professional to uncover their causes. The process may well bring you to an important evaluation of your previous years of life, one in which you experience the "death" of what has gone before. As in the loss of someone close to you, you may need to work through your grief over that loss, moving through shock and grief to recovery.

The butterfly is the Mexican spiritual symbol of the soul for this very good reason: the old life form must pass away before the new form takes flight in harmony and beauty. Allow yourself to cocoon and renew if that is what you need. Consider trying the following supportive tonics and other healing herbs. Pay attention to lifestyle changes, rather than short-circuiting the symptoms with mood-altering substances such as alcohol or even continued estrogen therapy, or overuse of antidepressant drugs. Antidepressants can prevent suicidal mood swings with or without menopausal symptoms, but in my opinion they are too commonly prescribed. If you are not sure whether or not you need Lyrica, Prozac, or the latest offering from Big Pharma that you have been prescribed, first, read up about them. Look at more than one or two websites or texts. Second, seek a second opinion. Finally, you must choose what is best for you.

Herbal Medicine

The following formulas use menopausal remedies with complementary properties to ease nagging aches and depression; these include black cohosh (*Cimicifuga racemosa*), wild yam root (*Dioscorea villosa*), and St. John's wort (*Hypericum perforatum*). Many of these *nervines* (herbs benefiting the nerves) have an affinity for encouraging healthy reproductive function. Used together, damiana (*Turnera diffusa*) and black cohosh relax muscles, lessen pain, calm the nerves, and strengthen the body. This combined benefit often enables women to cope better with all the taxing changes of dealing with self-image and sexuality during menopause. For example, the long-term use of St. John's wort has been found to be successful in helping women come off antidepressants such as Valium. For an antidepressant effect, it should be used for a minimum of eight weeks. Weaning yourself off Valium is best done under the supervision of a qualified and sympathetic care provider who is familiar with both herbs and Valium. Black cohosh is contained in many standard European and American menopausal formulas because it helps normalize natural estrogen levels and reduce nervous tension. It has an affinity for decreasing joint pain and stabilizing mood swings; it also has the bonus effect of toning the lungs.

The following combinations are recommended for depression, emotional vulnerability, and nervous tension. Think of them as all-natural fuel for the little engine that says, "I think I can, I think I can." Though neither extract nor tea is a delightful-tasting beverage, one or both will lighten your mood while strengthening your power. If you wish, add honey or other delicious herbs (peppermint, fennel, hibiscus) to taste. If you have blood sugar problems, don't use sugar or more than 1 teaspoon of honey per cup.

Concentrate for nervous system support

CONCENTRATED HERB EXTRACT	ACTIONS
2 oz. St. John's wort herb *(Hypericum perforatum)*	Repairs nerve damage; acts as antidepressant
4 oz. eleuthero root *(Eleutherococcus senticosus)*	Improves response to stress
2 oz. peppermint leaf *(Mentha piperita)*	Aromatherapy lifts spirits; is cleansing and soothing to digestion
1 oz. vervain herb *(Verbena officinalis)*	Tones liver; balances mood, hormones
1 oz. licorice root *(Glycyrrhiza glabra)*	Moistening; anti-inflammatory

Combine the extracts. Take 1 teaspoon in 1 cup of water, juice, or any herb tea three times a day. For immediate help in coping with difficult times in the short term, take ½ teaspoon every fifteen to twenty minutes, up to a total of 3 teaspoons (six doses) in two hours, plus the usual 3 teaspoons per day, as needed. These higher amounts can be continued for a week or two, especially if a crisis is also being handled through spot counseling or other appropriate help. If vervain is not available, replace it with 1 ounce of skullcap (Scutellaria laterifolia). If water retention, high blood pressure, or flavor are a problem, replace licorice with rhodiola (Rhodiola rosea).

Ten ounces will last two weeks or more depending on need.

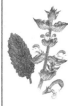

Tea for nervous system support

DRIED HERBS	ACTIONS
2¾ oz. damiana herb *(Turnera diffusa)*	Stimulates nerves and sluggish digestion
1 oz. raspberry leaf *(Rubus idaeus)*	Calming; nutritive; provides minerals; tones womb
1 oz. St. John's wort herb *(Hypericum perforatum)*	Antidepressant; improves resistance
3 oz. lemon balm leaf *(Melissa officinalis)*	For taste; improves digestion, mood
¼ oz. unsprayed/organic rose petals *(Rosa species)*	Tonic; astringent; for beauty

Combine ½ ounce of the mixture with 3 cups of boiling water in a teapot or container with a well-fitting lid. Let stand for fifteen minutes before straining. Drink 1 cup, hot or cold, three times a day. One teapot as strong as you like can be used as often as needed. Or, if you prefer, sip tea all day or drink two large glasses twice a day, making sure you drink 3 cups a day. Take for eight weeks or more for lasting benefits. If lemon balm or borage flowers are unavailable, replace with lemon verbena (a pleasant leaf from Peru, variously named Aloysia citriodora, Verbena triphylla, Verbena citriodora, Lippia triphylla, *or* Lippia citriodora*).*

Eight ounces will last two weeks.

Concentrate for emotional lows

CONCENTRATED HERB EXTRACT	ACTIONS
4 oz. passionflower herb *(Passiflora incarnata)*	Pain relieving; emotionally calming
2 oz. chamomile flower *(Matricaria recutita)*	Calming to nerves, digestion; reduces bloating and inflammation
1 oz. lemon balm leaf *(Melissa officinalis)*	Gladdens the heart
1 oz. violet flower *(Viola tricolor)*	Soothing; antioxidant; aromatic poetry

Combine these herbal extracts. Take 1 teaspoon in 1 cup of water, juice, or any herb tea in the morning and evening.

Eight ounces will last two weeks.

DRIED HERBS

3 oz. passionflower herb *(Passiflora incarnata)*

1 oz. sage leaf *(Salvia officinalis)*

1 oz. skullcap herb *(Scutellaria laterifolia)*

2 oz. chamomile flower *(Matricaria recutita)*

1 oz. cinnamon bark *(Cinnamomum species)*

ACTIONS

Pain relieving; emotionally calming

Supports hormonal balance, digestion; for taste

Nourishes; soothes nervous tension

Calming to nerves, digestion; reduces bloating

Warms and tones; astringent

Combine ½ ounce of the mixture with 3 cups of boiling water in a teapot or container with a well-fitting lid. Let stand for fifteen minutes before straining. Drink 1 cup, hot or cold, two to four times a day, or if you prefer, sip tea all day. If you are allergic to the daisy family, especially chrysanthemums, replace the chamomile with an extra ½ ounce of cinnamon and 1½ ounces of linden (Tilia species).

Eight ounces will last two weeks.

Nutrition

Review the following suggestions for whole foods that provide vitamins and minerals to address your mood, as well as the list of natural supplements.

wise food choices

❋ To improve liver metabolism, mood, and digestion, eat bitter, leafy vegetables, such as radicchio, endive, young dandelion greens, and kale. Also try edible flowers in salads, especially those in yellow-orange and blue-purple colors, such as spicy nasturtiums and sweet violets; these provide health-giving pigments, beta-carotene, and other nutrients.

❋ Avoid alcohol. Though it may feel good at first, it is a nerve depressant; it also interacts with estrogen activity and can damage the liver.

❋ Avoid caffeine and chocolate (even though there is an adrenaline rush, it hurts the nerves and eventually worsens the adrenal stress response).

supplements

❋ Use evening primrose oil, borage, or flaxseed, as directed on labels.

DYSMENORRHEA AND REPRODUCTIVE SYSTEM PAIN

Chronic pelvic pain and pelvic organ prolapse are more likely causes of pain in women at this age because fibroids usually improve with the menopausal drop in ovarian estrogen levels. Similarly, dysmenorrhea is less likely at this age. *Dysmenorrhea* is a catchall word meaning "painful or difficult menstrual bleeding." It can include cramps, painful arthritic inflammation, migraines, and pelvic pressure, perhaps with bloating or alternating diarrhea and constipation. A common symptom for both dysmenorrhea and prolapse is often described as a dragging sensation. This achiness may come with a feeling that the contents of the pelvis are being pulled downward. Chronic pelvic pain (CCP) in women is defined as pain below the navel for six months or longer. Chronic pelvic pain is a symptom rather than a disease. In one out five women the cause is gynecological, such as organ prolapse (connective tissue no longer supports the uterus as it once did), pelvic inflammatory disease (PID), or endometriosis. Other causes of chronic pelvic pain are located in the digestive tract, such as irritable bowel syndrome, or in the urinary tract (infection or interstitial cystitis). Fibromyalgia (chronic pain from an array of causes) or even problems with blood vessels in the pelvis have been at the bottom of some cases of CPP. In many women, though, the cause of CPP is never found. Treatments depend on the cause. Relaxation, meditation, biofeedback, acupuncture, and herbal support have all been found to be helpful. For more information that is tailored to you specifically, ask your health care provider or read more at www.uptodate.com/patients. The symptoms of CPP involve the reproductive and the nervous systems. Used in conjunction with moderate exercise, a good diet, and abundant rest, the herbal remedy suggestions that follow promote circulation, strengthen nerves, eliminate congestion, and bring better tone to the ligaments.

Sometimes a woman's pain threshold shifts around this time of the month and during the perimenopausal period. Because pain of any kind is an important message, the combinations in this section are designed so they will not suppress symptoms, but they are strong enough to take the edge off pain and provide some emergency relief. They can be used once or twice as needed for minor symptoms or for one to three months for more longstanding conditions. It takes at least ninety days for natural remedies to make significant improvements in chronic conditions. If symptoms don't feel minor to you, always know that a caring licensed health-care practitioner can rule out problems requiring more immediate attention.

Herbal Medicine

Concentrate for pelvic pain

CONCENTRATED HERB EXTRACT

4 oz. passionflower herb *(Passiflora incarnata)*

4 oz. cramp bark *(Viburnum opulus)*

2 oz. valerian root *(Valeriana officinalis)*

ACTIONS

Pain relieving; emotionally calming

Relaxes muscle spasms; relieves pain from tension

Sedates; relieves spasms; induces sleepiness

Combine these herbal extracts. For pain relief right now, start with ten drops every five minutes for twenty minutes. If that doesn't help, take ½ ounce diluted in ½ cup water, and sip over the next twenty minutes. Repeat as needed.

   Ten ounces will last thirty days.

If you experience chronic dull or aching pain before, after, or during your period, take ½ teaspoon in water three times every day for three weeks before the next period and during the flow if needed. If your cycle is erratic, so that "three weeks before" is impossible to predict, you can safely use the mixture all through the month and during the flow. Note that some people react to valerian with the opposite effect of insomnia; if you feel any increased agitation, replace the valerian with corydalis extract.

Tea for pelvic pain

DRIED HERBS

4 oz. passionflower herb *(Passiflora incarnata)*

3 oz. blackhaw root bark *(Viburnum prunifolium)*

2 oz. sage leaf *(Salvia officinalis)*

½ oz. ginger root *(Zingiber officinale)*

ACTIONS

Pain reliving; emotionally calming

Relaxes ovarian, uterine muscle spasms

Supports hormonal balance, digestion; for taste

Improves circulation, metabolism; for taste

Combine ⅓ ounce of the mixture with 3 cups of boiling water in a teapot or container with a well-fitting lid. Let stand for fifteen minutes before straining. Drink 2 cups, hot or cold, as needed.

   Fifteen ounces will last about thirty days.

Painful intercourse caused by dysmenorrhea, fibroids, or loss of lubrication in the vaginal canal is also associated with menopause. Though sex helps all these conditions, it is hard to have good sex when it doesn't feel good. Many herbs are known to help women's enjoyment of sexuality by healing, toning, and calming inflamed vaginal tissue, lubricating thin walls, or relaxing taut muscles. For example, wound-healing herbs such as yarrow (*Achillea millefolium*) and calendula (*Calendula officinalis*) are toning and anti-inflammatory when used directly on vaginal tissues. They are particularly beneficial if pain is caused by dryness, infection, or irritation. The following herb formulas relieve pain while healing from the inside out; also see the recommendations in "Vaginal Thinning and Dryness" (page 78).

Taken internally in tea form or as extracts, many of these same herbs are also digestive bitters. This is nature's way of feeding two birds with one morsel: hormonal and digestive changes are treated together. From the inside of the body, herbs can help relieve pelvic congestion, sluggish bowels, bloating, intestinal gas, and even heavy menstrual flow. Other digestive herbs with helpful properties for improving the integrity of the vaginal walls and uterine muscle during menopause are sage (*Salvia officinalis*), licorice (*Glycyrrhiza glabra*), and chamomile (*Matricaria recutita*).

Different types of pain respond to different herbs. Many common types of pain related to menopause can respond to the following two combinations. These remedies work on hormonal balance, sensory nerve endings, and adrenal stress. They also improve pelvic congestion and satisfactory elimination by activating the liver rather than stimulating the wall of the colon. This makes them milder, safer, and more comfortable to use than fast-acting herbal laxatives such as senna. *Cascara sagrada*, senna pods, and other strong anthraquinone-containing herbs are still useful in a pinch for constipation, but they work only on a symptomatic level and can be harsh on the body. The digestive bitter tonics used here are better for balancing sluggish or congested bowels in conjunction with bloating, gas, or even some alternating looseness of stools. If there's nothing wrong with the digestive tract, these herbs are mild enough to not overstimulate elimination. The combination will still offer its pain-lessening and nourishing qualities. When our mood changes we tend to develop inflammation, while inflammatory pain may be a background trigger for feeling depressed.

If you need to sleep to give your body a chance to escape constant or chronic pain, use the following herb as a last resort for quick symptom relief:

VALERIAN CONCENTRATED HERB EXTRACT

1 oz. valerian root *(Valeriana officinalis)*

ACTIONS

Pain relieving; sedates; relaxes muscle tension

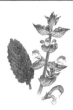

Dilute ten to fifteen drops of this pungent root extract in water, juice, or herb tea and take every ten to fifteen minutes until pain is gone. This usually occurs in two or three doses; don't take more than ten doses in any two-hour period. By that point, sleep will be on the horizon anyway. A tea of the root, ½ ounce to 1 pint of water, is also effective, though it doesn't taste good and smells peculiar; drink a teacup at a time as needed. Nonalcohol extracts with glycerin are available in many stores and taste better but are slightly less effective.

Note: *Some people react to valerian with increased agitation and sleeplessness. If this occurs with you, discontinue and try breathing, visualization, and simple chamomile tea.*

Yet another cause of pain is the menstrual migraine. This form of headache also may flare up in menopause and is aggravated by excess estrogen, caffeine, and other factors. Prevention is the best remedy for these headaches, whether they are related to the menstrual cycle or changing estrogen levels in menopause. Prevention includes eating regularly to stabilize blood sugar, releasing tension before it builds up, and taking herbs to ease premenstrual or menopausal irritability. When it is too late for prevention, try one or more of the following three remedies to feel an immediate difference. There are three choices because each will not work for every woman, and you may need to experiment to get the relief you need. As we age, we are all at increased risk for stroke and cerebral bleeds. These events are not usually confused with migraine. If you have head pain that you cannot explain, see a care provider. Also, if you have a family history, a personal history, or more than a few risk factors for stroke, any needed changes in lifestyle are now considered the best prevention.

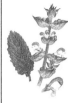

Concentrate for cerebral circulation

CONCENTRATED HERB EXTRACT	ACTIONS
2 oz. butterbur *(Petasites hybridus)*	Anti-inflammatory; specific to head pain
2 oz. skullcap herb *(Scutellaria laterifolia)*	Relaxes tension, anxiety; nourishes nerves
2 oz. lavender flower *(Lavandula officinalis)*	Cleanses; relaxes; lifts spirits
2 oz. motherwort herb *(Leonurus cardiaca)*	Lowers tension and high blood pressure

Combine these herbal extracts. Take 1 to 3 teaspoons in 1 cup of water, juice, or any herb tea up to ten times a day if needed. At maximum dose, that's 30 teaspoons or just over 4 ounces in a day, so be sure to drink plain water and other fluids, eat small meals, and rest. If your headache requires that much tincture, avoid driving; instead, stay home or take a stress-relieving walk.

Eight ounces will last a long time without refrigeration; keep on hand for occasional headaches.

Tea for cerebral circulation

DRIED HERBS	ACTIONS
3 oz. gotu kola leaf, herb *(Centella asiatica)*	Specific tea to nourish nerves; antioxidant; anti-inflammatory
2 oz. skullcap herb *(Scutellaria laterifolia)*	Reduces pressure, tension
2 oz. linden flower *(Tilia* species*)*	Reduces high blood pressure; calms; moistens
½ oz. rosemary flower, leaf *(Rosmarinus officinalis)*	Relaxes blood vessels
½ oz. sage leaf *(Salvia officinalis)*	Supports hormonal balance; tonic; astringent

Combine ½ ounce of the mixture with 3 cups of boiling water in a teapot or container with a well-fitting lid. Let stand for five to fifteen minutes before straining. Drink 2 cups hot or cold, as needed. To improve flavor, add plain water or Rooibos herb tea to taste.

Eight ounces stored in a closed container away from direct heat and light will last up to a year without refrigeration.

If you experience menstrual migraines, which are caused by blood vessel spasms, prevention is even more necessary than for tension headaches. The best herbal remedies for this type of head-ache do not get rid of a migraine once you have it; rather, they build up your resistance to future headaches. The main extract, feverfew (*Chrysanthemum parthenium*), must be made from the fresh flowering herb because dried tea has far less of an effect. Most companies know this; check the label of any store-bought extract to be sure it is from fresh plant material. Some women report that freeze-dried capsules work; others report they do not. When you feel like closing the door, disconnecting the phone, or heading for the hills, do that and also take a cup of the following remedy.

Concentrate for migraines

CONCENTRATED HERB EXTRACT	ACTIONS
3 oz. fresh feverfew herb (*Chrysanthemum parthenium*)	Stabilizes blood vessels to brain
2 oz. chaste berry seed (*Vitex agnus-castus*)	Stabilizes hormones
1 oz. lavender flower (*Lavandula officinalis*)	Cleanses; relaxes; uplifts
2 oz. sage leaf (*Salvia officinalis*)	Tonic; astringent; supports hormonal balance

Initially, take 1 teaspoon diluted in 1 cup of liquid every morning for a minimum of sixty days; to mask its odd taste, try it in diluted fruit juice or herb tea. Take an extra dose if you feel a migraine sneaking up on you. Do not stop this suddenly, or a rebound migraine will be more likely. Taper down to ½ teaspoon every morning for another three weeks, then ¼ teaspoon for an additional three weeks, then ¼ teaspoon every other day for another three weeks. At this point, keep the blend on hand, avoiding any known triggers other than menses.

Eight ounces will last up to a year out of direct light and heat and can be used as needed.

When all is said and done, pain is sometimes not just physical or just emotional. When you know the cause of severe pain, but it has not responded to the gentle methods just described, it is not wrong or weak to suppress it. Allowing yourself escape routes in severe distress can allow your body's resources to mobilize for deep healing. The use of nature's painkillers can also contribute to healing in this way.

When physical or emotional pain is severe, take up to 1 ounce of passionflower tincture diluted in one 8-ounce cup of water or herb tea. If pain in your lower back or abdomen is causing insomnia, try massaging the affected area with the aromatherapy blend noted under "In Addition," page 67. Or take a lavender bath or even a warm shower that ends with a lukewarm or cool rinse. Then return to bed with a cup of sleep-inducing herb tea. This can be the formula called "Tea for restorative sleep" (page 138), in chapter 4, or a single herb, from mild chamomile to medium-strong motherwort (very bitter tasting) to the stronger valerian (strong tasting). Of these, only the chamomile tastes good as a tea to most women, so other useful forms are capsules (which may take up to an hour and a half to take effect) or glycerin tinctures, which have no alcohol. Alcohol-based tinctures work as well, but if you need to avoid alcohol (even a small amount of alcohol can trigger migraines in some women), do not use them.

The amount of alcohol in herbal extracts is relatively little when taken as directed, so if a small quantity of alcohol is not a problem for you, you can, of course, use alcohol-based tinctures. It is the herb, not the alcohol, that is having the effect, so you are not really using the tincture as a stiff snort, as some skeptics might scoff. If you are in great pain, it will not help to sip 1 to 3 teaspoons of Scotch diluted in a cup of water before bed. However, this dose or less of the herb extracts can work wonders. This way of using herbs is not to be repeated long term, but it does work well for short-term symptom management of pain or insomnia.

The purpose of using these particular pain-lessening herb formulas is not to suppress each symptom but to improve the quality of life *in the moment* while we are still working on the causes of our discomfort. Returning to sleep in itself allows deeper self-healing, even if the sleep is achieved on some nights with repeated doses of valerian. Remember, we are still discussing strong plant preparations, not habit-forming pharmaceutical drugs.

Nutrition

Review the following suggestions for whole foods that provide vitamins and minerals to address reproductive system pain.

wise food choices

❀ Avoid animal fats, including dairy and goat cheese, because they form prostaglandins, a large group of powerful hormonelike compounds that act locally on blood vessels, pain receptors, and a wide range of life processes. Prostaglandins from animal protein and fat lower the pain threshold, worsening painful cramping. (One type of prostaglandins worsens pain and inflammation, whereas other prostaglandins have totally opposite and even unrelated effects.)

❀ Drink plain water for all kinds of headaches.

❀ Eat a piece of fruit or a small meal to alleviate stress headaches or raise low blood sugar, which may itself cause headaches or worsen the stress response.

❀ If you have painful periods with heavy flow and clotting, eat more carrots; drink 8 ounces of carrot juice a day for ten days before each cycle to lessen clotting.

In Addition

❀ To help relieve headaches, close your eyes for fifteen minutes.

❀ For headaches, especially when you are tired, massage just five to ten drops of essential oil of lavender and/or rosemary into the temples and the back of the neck.

❀ For stress, if you have time, add five to ten drops of lavender or chamomile essential oil to a relaxing bath.

Aromatherapy blend for pain

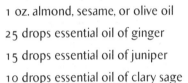

1 oz. almond, sesame, or olive oil

25 drops essential oil of ginger

15 drops essential oil of juniper

10 drops essential oil of clary sage

Combine the essential oils with almond, sesame, or olive oil. Massage into painful lower back, thighs, and buttocks and down backs of legs. Repeat as often as needed. Use externally only. If skin sensitivity develops, discontinue use and wash with cool water and a mild soap; pat dry.

HOT FLASHES AND NIGHT SWEATS

In Great Britain and Australia, hot flashes are known as *flushing*. For the longest time, I thought it was their accent, but they really do say, "Poor dear, she's having a hot flush." For many women, hot flashes are no joke. They can be the most debilitating symptom of menopause, though they can improve or even disappear through natural means. A hot flash is a sudden sensation of heat from blood vessels near the skin, sometimes with profuse sweating and sometimes preceded by chills. A hot flash starts in the chest and rises up the neck and face, and though it happens from head to toe, it is felt most in the upper body. Hot flashes that occur at night, especially with more perspiration, are called *night sweats*. Generally, women who build up their health can soften the negative symptoms of hot flashes, some reporting that hot flashes become so minor that they are felt as pleasurable little waves.

When a hot flash occurs, what is happening in your body? The hot flash begins in the hypothalamus, a part of the brain. Among other things, the hypothalamus controls body temperature and, through feedback from the body, regulates estrogen levels. When estrogen starts to drop in an uneven stop-and-start style, as frequently happens during menopause, the hypothalamus sends a chemical messenger—gonadotropin-releasing hormone, or GNRH—to the pituitary gland. The GNRH tells the pituitary to send follicle-stimulating hormone (FSH) to the ovaries; in turn, FSH politely requests the ovaries to hurry up with some estrogen by stimulating an egg follicle to develop with its usual yield of ovarian estrogen. The ovaries will or won't respond to this stimulus, depending on their ability to do so. Around menopause the ovaries may not have enough viable eggs left.

If an egg follicle develops under the influence of FSH, the estrogen it produces builds up to a certain level. Then this higher level of estrogen gives feedback to the brain to stop sending out FSH. If there is no viable egg left to develop, there is no ovulation, so there is no high buildup of estrogen, so there is no feedback to the brain. The result? The pituitary in the brain causes FSH to soar, trying to meet the usual goal of stimulating increased estrogen by repeating itself more loudly.

So what now? If the ovary cannot comply with the usual orders from the brain, the body responds to low estrogen by trying to storm the hypothalamus with adrenaline to get it moving. This tempest in a teapot affects the hypothalamus's temperature-control center, resetting the body's thermostat control for heat to reach a higher temperature, as if you were turning up the thermostat on your home's heating system. During a hot flash, you may actually feel a little chill before your body temperature feels hot-hot-hot in comparison to the new setting. The heart rate responds to the adrenaline's effect on the hypothalamus by speeding up a little or a lot, depending on the woman or the strength of each particular hot flash. All the blood vessels, from the heart to the skin, dilate, allowing the body to cool by evaporation and bringing the temperature down to the new temperature set by the hypothalamus.

Hot flashes are triggered by stress, any form of heat (a tense office meeting, the weather outside, too many covers on the bed, a lover's body in bed), and "vasodilators"—substances that dilate the blood vessels: hot coffee, capsaicin (the substance that makes chile peppers spicy hot), and alcohol. Though nicotine causes blood vessels to contract, smoking also worsens hot flashes. Even menopause itself makes the blood vessels more vulnerable to temperature signals. Our blood vessels are more sensitive to drops and surges in estrogen and other hormones at this time. The body's feedback system notices all this flurry and checks to see why the temperature control was reset. After days, weeks, or months, your body gets tired of playing this exciting game, and figures out how to be at peace with its lower levels of estrogen. The time range varies widely from woman to woman. The feedback system has tried all its usual controls and finally sees that this is no temporary glitch. It is time for a new state of hormone balance. It is time for a Change.

Because women's blood vessels become more sensitive to sharp drops and floods of chemicals, including hormones, during the Change, the objective of taking certain herbs at this time is twofold: to stabilize blood vessel sensitivity to changing hormone levels, and to slow down or smooth the overall drop in estrogen from the ovaries. Some of these herbs do this by supporting the adrenal function. Our adrenals provide a little estrogen as a hormonal cushion. Adrenal tonic herbs, called *adaptogens*, help our adrenal glands help us *adapt* to current levels of stress. Examples are nettle (*Urtica dioica*), eleuthero (*Eleutherococcus senticosus*), borage (*Borago officinalis*), and ginseng (*Panax ginseng*). Though some herbalists find that ginseng is too heating for women with hot flashes, clinical trials of women using moderately low doses of *Panax* ginseng find it relieves vasomotor symptoms such as night sweats and hot flashes. Nervines are another category of herbs that do more than simply suppress hot flashes: they help the body handle stress by providing relaxation, stimulation, or pain relief. They can mitigate hot flashes because, as every woman knows from experience and recent research has shown, the endocrine (hormone) and nervous systems are not two separate systems—each improves or worsens depending on the health or strain on the other. Nourishing herbs like motherwort (*Leonurus cardiaca*) that calm frazzled nerve endings can help make hot flashes disappear or at least be more comfortable (in severe cases, more tolerable).

One particular herb or another in this section may relieve hot flashes time and again for some women. But for severe or stubborn hot flashes, more women find better results from combinations of herbs that support the liver's natural function of metabolizing circulating hormones and the estrogen still made in our bodies. Wisely combined formulas also optimize the function of all types of estrogen, from ovaries, adrenal glands, and even fat cells. Hormonal tonics such as licorice (*Glycyrrhiza glabra*) can do double duty by optimizing liver function and acting on the adrenal glands as a nourishing tonic.

Night sweats and palpitations (feeling your heart pound) can be addressed with herbal cardiovascular tonics, nervine relaxants, and hormonal balancers such as dong quai (*Angelica sinensis*), motherwort (*Leonurus cardiaca*), linden (*Tilia platyphylla/T. europea*), and yarrow (*Achillea millefolium*). These four plants, used singly or in any combination, stabilize the sensitivity of blood vessels to ebbs and flows in estrogen. The following two formulas strengthen and tone the blood vessels and, through the addition of hormone balancers such as chaste berry (*Vitex agnus-castus*), normalize your system's changing amounts of estrogen. Taken as a tea or concentrate, black cohosh (*Cimicifuga racemosa*) has milder but broader effects than extracts or proprietary products such as Remifemin. Tea or capsule dose is 1 gram of dried root three times a day.

It often takes six weeks or even as long as twelve months of treatment to decrease symptoms such as night sweats to a manageable level. Herbalists usually prescribe whole plant extracts of black cohosh in combination with other herbs over the course of many months before tapering off gradually, while monitoring to avoid early signs of sensitivity (frontal headache, temporary GI upset).

Herbal Medicine

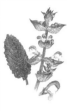

Concentrate for keeping cool

CONCENTRATED HERB EXTRACT	ACTIONS
2 oz. black cohosh root (*Cimicifuga racemosa*)	Reduces luteinizing hormone; thought to be linked to hot flashes
2 oz. motherwort herb (*Leonurus cardiaca*)	Directs peripheral blood to digestion; cools symptoms; calms heart palpitations
2 oz. hawthorn flower, leaf, berry (*Crataegus species*)	Protects heart; strengthens blood vessels against hormonal ebbs and flows
2 oz. yarrow flower (*Achillea millefolium*)	Cools temperature; stimulates liver
1 oz. chaste berry seed (*Vitex agnus-castus*)	Stabilizes drops and surges in progesterone and, indirectly, estrogens
1 oz. sage leaf (*Salvia officinalis*)	Reduces sweating

Combine these herbal extracts. Every ten minutes take one dropper or ¼ teaspoon diluted in ¼ cup of room-temperature water. This remedy usually works in two or three doses, but the effect won't last long unless you take it consistently. For more permanent improvement, take 1 teaspoon three times a day for two weeks, take a few days off, then repeat for another two weeks. After that, repeat as needed.

Ten ounces will last thirty days.

This concentrate combines well with the tea described next. The "cucumber" in the tea is really borage, a flowering edible plant whose peeled stalk smells and tastes a little like cucumbers. The overall effect of this tea is stabilizing, soothing, and moistening.

Tea for keeping cool

DRIED HERBS	ACTIONS
2 oz. linden flower *(Tilia* species*)*	Relaxes nerves; lowers high blood pressure
2 oz. borage flowers, stems, and leaves *(Borago officinalis)*	Moistens; nutritive tonic
2 oz. hibiscus flower *(Hibiscus sabdariffa)*	Cooling; for taste
1 oz. marshmallow root *(Althaea officinalis)*	Moistens; helps water balance
1 oz. chamomile flower *(Matricaria recutita)*	Soothes stomach, nerves

Combine 1 ounce of the mixture with 3 cups of boiling water in a teapot or container with a well-fitting lid. Let stand for fifteen minutes, then strain the tea and store it in a closed container. Allow to cool; drink at room temperature–not hot and not icy cold. During daytime hot flashes, drink 1 cup as often as needed, or, if you prefer, sip this amount of tea all day or drink two large glasses twice a day–just be sure you drink it all sometime each day. The tea is also good for sipping while you are drying off from a cool bath or shower. Drink ½ to 3 cups as needed after night sweats before you return to a fresh, dry bed, but remember to empty your bladder before going to sleep.

Eight ounces will last two weeks.

Nutrition

Review the following suggestions for whole foods that provide vitamins and minerals to address hot flashes and night sweats, as well as the list of natural supplements.

wise food choices

❀ Choose foods that are high in vitamin C. Among the many options are citrus fruits; rosehip jam (although vitamin C is lost in cooking except in some high-quality brands, natural fruit pectins and bioflavonoids offer fiber and other benefits to vessel tone); fresh, raw, green sweet bell peppers; fresh, raw broccoli (raw broccoli is high in vitamin C; lightly steamed or stir-fried is OK).

❀ Avoid cayenne pepper and other hot spices. Cayenne may seem like a good food source of vitamin C, but stimulating spices aggravate hot flashes, causing blood vessels at the skin's surface to open up and evaporate the heat; the resulting perspiration cools down the body. Though I encourage women to incorporate garlic into their regular way of eating because of its many health benefits, some women with sensitivity to onions and garlic find it triggers their unique pattern of heat symptoms.

❀ Avoid caffeine (including soft drinks, chocolate, and aspirin containing caffeine) and alcohol.

❀ Great alternatives to the supplements listed next are home-sprouted seeds and nuts, rich in essential fatty acids, proteins, and enzymes, and easy for menopausal women to assimilate.

❀ Also highly recommended are foods rich in natural plant estrogens (phytoestrogens) that augment our own estrogen, such as soy flour, red clover sprouts, and flaxseeds. For more information about these foods, see the sidebar "Herbs and Nutrition in Menopause" starting on page 37.

supplements

❀ Some women find that 600 to 800 I.U. (international units) of vitamin E taken daily is useful for hot flashes. For better metabolism of dosages higher than 600 I.U., you can add 1 to 3 grams of vitamin C (1,000 to 3,000 milligrams) and divide the mixture into three equal doses. For example, in the morning, at midday, and in the evening, you would take 200 I.U. of vitamin E with 1 gram of C. After a week you should be able to reduce your intake of vitamin E to 400 I.U. daily. But please know that more is *not* better! It is best not to take more than 1,200 I.U. daily in long-term use. The conservative recommended limit is 100 I.U. daily if you have diabetes, hypertension, or a rheumatic heart condition.

❀ Evening primrose oil in capsules is also effective for hot flashes. Most research suggests the minimum dose in a range of 3 to 5 grams a day, represented by six to ten capsules of 500 milligrams each. It may be effective as quickly as three to six weeks. For sensitive women, even two to four capsules a day may help.

❀ Motherwort metabolizes fats and hormones, filters blood, and improves immunity. It is specifically helpful for heart palpitations as well as menopausal hot flashes and healthy liver function, so it may be useful in any formula taken by a woman with cardiovascular concerns. Dosage of store-bought extract ranges from one dropperful to 1 teaspoon every ten to twenty minutes as needed and/or three times a day for prevention.

❀ Ginseng (*Panax ginseng*, also called Asian, Chinese, Korean, or Manchurian ginseng) taken for six weeks and longer works well too, although it may not work equally well in all women. Some traditional Chinese medical practitioners say that menopausal women should never take ginseng. Nevertheless, numerous women have told me of the benefits it gave them, and there is research to support both views. Those women who seem to react badly to ginseng are generally, to begin with, tired but high-strung, tense, and wound up, whereas women who do well with a little ginseng tend to feel, before taking the herb, emptied out, weakened in every body system, and slow to get going. The use of ginseng is certainly easier on a woman than HRT. The temporary "ginseng headache" that helps a person determine that this powerful herb may not be right for her is not as difficult a side effect to clear up as the cancer risk associated with replacement hormones.

❀ Licorice is a rich, affordable source of phytoestrogens. Although it should be used with some caution, moderate amounts or the conservative dosages suggested in this book are going to be helpful to most women going through the Change. An explanation of precautions is found in "Irregular Cycles," which follows. Formulas including this herb also indicate substitutes.

❀ Natural sources of phytoestrogens commonly available in herb shops or natural-food stores require a different kind of caution. Sarsaparilla is sometimes adulterated (mixed with other herb substitutes), so ask to make sure you are buying pure Jamaican sarsaparilla—*Smilax ornata* or a related *Smilax* species. Real sarsaparilla has little fragrance; the more delicious the smell, the more likely it is to be a different plant that confusingly also bears the common name of sarsaparilla. Because of rampant overharvesting, do not purchase the endangered wild American ginseng (*Panax quinquefolium*). Please use only cultivated roots, grown and harvested with ecological sensitivity.

In Addition

❀ If you are having sudden hot flashes, wear light layers of cotton clothing. And no turtlenecks! During a hot flash, try leaving the room for a change of scene or loosening your collar.

❀ Because hot flashes and sweating often worsen at night, you may want to open windows before bedtime if it is safe and practical to do so.

❀ Night sweats can drench a bed, so invest in two sets of cotton or linen bedding, and keep the extra set and other comfortable bedding at hand. Women report that imagining that day's problems confined to the pile of damp sheets wadded on the floor, destined for tomorrow's laundry, is helpful to them. If you feel the need to shower, wash in warm water and end with cooler water. Cooling off after a warm shower sends blood from peripheral vessels back to the interior of the body, indirectly resulting in a neuronal message directing your body to get drowsy. Keep a thermos or other container of tea for bedtime (see chapter 4, "Postmenopause") in a convenient place nearby to further help you get back to sleep.

Though all this may seem like an undue amount of nighttime activity when you are fatigued, these steps help you focus your attention on returning to a comfortable bed for a few more hours of real sleep, instead of tossing about in a damp bed and drinking ever-stronger sleep-inducing herbs without the desired effect. I do not normally recommend strong "knock-out" herbs to get to sleep or return to sleep; rather, women do well when they accept that there may be a temporary break in sleep. Many report that an attitude of calm acceptance allows the disturbance to be minimized in the mind, and thus minimized in fact.

IRREGULAR CYCLES

First you have a late period. Then you have two in just six weeks. You haven't had one in six months, and you think, "Hey, that was easy!" but the next month there's a scarlet stain on your white sheets. When your biological clock starts winding down, your cycle becomes irregular and your emotions may well become unpredictable. This could be mildly annoying or it could be pelvic cancer, which is why every woman in menopause with unexpected bleeding should be evaluated.

The best way you can cope is to really take care of yourself. Deeply focus on stabilizing your body: prolong your naturally occurring estrogen levels, build your health, look beyond symptoms that come and go, nourish each of the body systems affected by the Change. Focus your inner being by drawing more love to yourself in your personal, social, and spiritual relationships. Tall order? Your energy and your spirit are limitless.

And nature offers some kind assistance. One or more of the hormonal normalizers found in every habitat on Earth, such as the North American black cohosh, support a grace-filled Change, as does chaste berry (*Vitex agnus-castus*), a Mediterranean seed in human use as a hormonal tonic for more than three thousand years.

China introduced dong quai (*Angelica sinensis*) root to the West, but my Euro-American tradition favors the use of chaste berry. In Europe, older herbal practitioners with whom I did my internship swore they could not treat menopause safely and effectively without this pungent seed. It may be that during other decades in the twentieth century, herbal alternatives such as American ginseng, red clover, and the cohoshes were not as fresh or high quality as chaste berry. Chinese herbs used for women in menopause, such as dong quai, bupleurum (*Bupleurum chinense*), and other companion herbs, were relatively unknown to Euro-American herbal traditions until recent years. False unicorn (*Chamaelirium luteum*), the root of which was once a standard American remedy, is endangered in the wild, so ethical herbal practitioners will not use it unless they personally collect it where it is locally abundant, even though it is still recommended in mass-produced herb books and formulas. Nature is generous in giving us several equally good herbs in the hormone-balancing category, so if we do not wish to destroy the plants we know and love, let us be equally generous in returning a little of our time to nature.

Herbal Medicine

Compared to the formulas to maintain menses naturally in chapter 1, the following two concentrates and tea are more nourishing for women in menopause. For irregular cycles complicated by heavy flow or for spotting between cycles, these are stronger than the herbal combinations given in chapter 1 for premenopausal women who are spotting. For the quickest results, this first formula works with the power of the moon's pull on gravity to establish a regular menses, even if it is not twenty-eight days. If your cycles have been erratic for longer than six months, or if you experience heavier flows (flooding), use the second formula or the tea version that follows instead.

Concentrate for nourishing reproductive support

CONCENTRATED HERB EXTRACT	ACTIONS
2 oz. black cohosh root (*Cimicifuga racemosa*)	Reduces tension; positive perimenopausal effects on bone and immune health
2 oz. chaste berry seed (*Vitex agnus-castus*)	Regulates pituitary control of hormones, especially luteinizing hormone and prolactin
2 oz. nettle leaf (*Urtica dioica*)	Nutritive; supports liver, kidney function
2 oz. bacopa herb (*Bacopa monniera*)	Improves mind-body function, memory, mood

Combine these herbal extracts. Take 1 teaspoon in 1 cup of water, juice, or any herb tea three times a day, morning, afternoon (3 to 5 PM) and after dinner. Though it may bring improvement in the first month, take for a minimum of three months for better results.

Eight ounces will last two weeks.

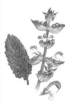

Concentrate for heavy, irregular flows

CONCENTRATED HERB EXTRACT	ACTIONS
2 oz. fresh shepherd's purse herb (*Capsella bursa-pastoris*)	Stops or slows excess bleeding
2 oz. lady's mantle leaf (*Alchemilla vulgaris*)	Astringent; protects reproductive tissue
1 oz. cinnamon bark (*Cinnamomum species*)	Astringent; warming
1 oz. blue cohosh root (*Caulophyllum thalictroides*)	Astringent; increases blood flow to reproductive organs in nonpregnant women; improves muscle health
1 oz. black cohosh root (*Cimicifuga racemosa*)	Reduces pain and some hormonal imbalance; relaxes

Note: *Both black and blue cohosh are contraindicated in pregnancy for any layperson; their use requires rigorous professional training and clinical experience. A perimenopausal woman with irregular periods is unlikely to be pregnant, but it is possible. If in doubt, leave these out or seek the advice of a professional herbalist (see Resources).*

Combine these extracts; take 1 to 3 teaspoons every two hours until flow stops or slows down. For chronic problems with spotting between cycles, flooding, and fibroids, see a health professional and, if appropriate, take 1 teaspoon three times a day for a minimum of three months (15 ounces per month). The main ingredient, shepherd's purse, is a mustard family member that tastes plain old bad. Get it down anyway. Put your legs up. Let it work.

Seven ounces will last approximately a week; this amount lasts three days or so if the higher dose is needed for short-term results.

DRIED HERBS	ACTIONS
3 oz. partridge berry herb *(Mitchella repens)*	Lessens excess flow; tones
3 oz. lady's mantle herb *(Alchemilla vulgaris)*	Protects reproductive tissues
1 oz. sage leaf *(Salvia officinalis)*	Astringent
1 oz. cinnamon bark *(Cinnamonum zeylanicum)*	For taste; soothes; lessens flow

Add 1 ounce of the mixture to 4 cups of boiling water in a teapot or container with a well-fitting lid. Let stand for fifteen minutes before straining. Drink 1 cup, hot or cold, three or four times a day. Or, if you prefer, sip tea all day or drink two large glasses twice a day, but make sure you drink 3 or 4 cups of tea in a day.

Eight ounces will last two weeks.

Nutrition

Review the following suggestions for whole foods that provide vitamins and minerals to address irregular cycles, as well as the list of natural supplements.

wise food choices

❀ In early spring, eat dandelion leaf in salads or mixed steamed greens.

❀ Try pomegranate seeds.

❀ Eat dried apricots as a snack.

❀ Try sesame seeds or tahini (1 tablespoon plain or in prepared dishes, two or three times a week).

supplements

❀ Milk thistle (1 tablespoon of seeds daily, ground into powder and sprinkled over cooked grains and salads or blended in soups). May be taken as capsules: two capsules three times a day or three capsules two times a day with meals. Standardized silymarin from milk thistle is also available; take as labels suggest.

❀ Beta-carotene obtained from yellow or orange vegetables is better than from supplements.

VAGINAL THINNING AND DRYNESS

During perimenopause and menopause, hormonal imbalance may thin or dry the lining of your vagina, causing it to become inflamed or sensitive. If you are experiencing discomfort during intercourse or if vaginal dryness persists despite sexual desire, you may have this condition, called *atrophic vaginitis*. To resolve it, you can take herbs to maximize the body's existing estrogen levels from the metabolism of androstenedione produced by the adrenal glands and stored in fat under the skin. Herbal remedies can also optimize progesterone, which helps maintain the necessary balance of sex hormones to keep vaginal tissue healthy. At the same time, you can use herbal remedies to restore the normal, helpful bacterial flora to the mucous membranes lining the vagina. Many of the plants that have this effect contain protective essential oils or other biochemicals that remove inappropriate microbes, with few of the side effects of drugs.

Last, but certainly not least, you can work to nourish a sense of emotional well-being within yourself. Vaginal dryness interferes with sex at a time when you may especially need the intimacy of sexual contact to weather challenges to your self-image and identity as a woman. But this condition does not mean your sex life is over: if you want to have sex, but you're already feeling friction or irritation, please know that you can have a moist vagina and pleasurable intercourse even long after the drop in estrogen that happens with menopause. All your hopes do not hang on estrogen alone. Women can have great sex beyond menopause if and when they want to. Yet another false stereotype is the one that libido (sex drive) goes down at menopause. For many, sex becomes a new adventure of body and soul. You may in fact find new appetites or paths to pleasure. But for many sex drive or vaginal lubrication does go down. This happens often enough to include natural remedies for women with diminished juice here.

In reality, women find that symptoms associated with hot flashes and vaginal dryness decrease with regular sex. Using sexual energy and releasing it through orgasm, as well as having a healthy attitude toward your changing body, are your best means of controlling the physical discomforts of menopause. Both sex shared with a partner and masturbation stimulate vaginal moisture and bring germ-fighting enzymes into the mucus produced by the glands in the vaginal wall. The blood flow from the head and heart all the way down to the pelvis from happy movements will help restore moisture and dynamic balance in the tissues.

Don't douche unless it helps relieve inflammation and seems absolutely necessary. In most instances you should not need to douche to sanitize or deodorize your vagina. When we are healthy inside our bodies, we are not dirty "down there." Strange odors or itches are a signal that an imbalance is blocking the self-cleaning ways of the body. Although vaginal applications may help symptoms such as dryness, thinning of the vaginal walls, or even the infections that may result from vaginal changes, douching without good reason may actually create more problems than it solves. One reason is that the repeated application of water is in itself eventually drying, making the thinner vaginal wall of menopause (already drier) even more susceptible to infections. Douching too much rinses away helpful lubrication, such as the enzyme-rich mucus that traps potential microbes. Douching also removes helpful bacterial flora that normally help us maintain an acidic vaginal secretion. This healthy vaginal environment prevents colonization of common opportunistic infections, including yeasts (*Candida*). Some healing vaginal applications are included in this section, but they are best used for short-term problems or in the context of other changes to clear up an existing condition.

Herbal Medicine

The following formulas prevent or minimize thinning of the vaginal lining by improving circulation, nutrition, and hormonal balance. These recipes utilize the multitalented phytoestrogenic herbs, which, arranged in different "bouquets," have slightly different effects. The following combinations may therefore resemble the recommendations in "Sexuality and Vaginal Changes," page 27, but they provide a more broad-based set of actions: they moisturize, strengthen, improve nonspecific immunity, and raise the spirits, especially those of the woman whose Change is well under way.

Concentrate for moistening tissues

CONCENTRATED HERB EXTRACT	ACTIONS
2 oz. wild yam root (*Dioscorea villosa*)	Anti-inflammatory; supports hormonal balance
2 oz. sarsaparilla root (*Smilax ornata*)	Supports lymph, immune, hormonal balance
1 oz. nettle leaf (*Urtica dioica*)	Nutritive; aids kidney, liver functions
2 oz. lady's mantle herb (*Alchemilla vulgaris*)	Protects and tones vaginal lining; supports hormonal balance
1 oz. ginger root (*Zingiber officinale*)	Improves and warms microcirculation

Combine these herbal extracts. Take 1 teaspoon in 1 cup of water, juice, or any herb tea in the morning and evening. You can take up to four times a day for quicker results. Best results may be seen after a minimum of two to three months.

Eight ounces will last about two weeks.

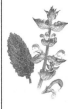

Tea for moistening tissues

DRIED HERBS	ACTIONS
3 oz. red clover flower *(Trifolium pratense)*	Phytoestrogens and minerals nourish tissues
2 oz. lady's mantle herb *(Alchemilla vulgaris)*	Tones, tightens vaginal lining
1¾ oz. marshmallow root *(Althaea officinalis)*	Improves flavor; adds moisture; nourishes tissues
1 oz. raspberry leaf *(Rubus idaeus)*	Provides calcium; calms nerves; tones tissues
¼ oz. licorice root *(Glycyrrhiza glabra)*	Moistens; aids digestion; anti-inflammatory

Add 1 ounce of the mixture to 3 or 4 cups of boiling water in a teapot or container with a well-fitting lid. Whole flowers of red clover are light and fluffy, so you may need 4 cups to cover the herbs. Let stand for fifteen minutes and then strain. Drink 1 cup, hot or cold, three times a day. Drinking a quart (4 cups) a day brings quicker results; best results are seen in two to three months.

Eight ounces will last about two weeks.

If you've had a chronic vaginal infection, this next herbal combination can be taken safely along with antibiotics, if those are considered necessary. Or this may be used to repair the immune system while preventing a recurrence or clearing up a vaginal infection. It especially helps after repeated courses of antibiotics, which are often prescribed for chronic conditions.

Concentrate for immune support

CONCENTRATED HERB EXTRACT	ACTIONS
2 oz. eleuthero root (*Eleutherococcus senticosus*)	Adaptogen; improves response to antimicrobials and antibiotics; reduces effects of stress on immune system
2 oz. St. John's wort herb (*Hypericum perforatum*)	Antiviral; nourishes nerves; antidepressant
2 oz. echinacea root (*Echinacea purpurea*)	Stimulates natural immunity and lymphatic function
2 oz. kava root (*Piper methysticum*)	Antimicrobial for the urinary tract; reduces painful spasms; safe at this dosage

Combine these herbal extracts. The kava tincture will make it cloudy, so shake well before each dose. It also tastes . . . bad. Stevia does not help here. Take 1 teaspoon in 1 cup of water, grape juice, or any strong-flavored herb tea (perhaps mint) every four hours for four days. Then reduce dosage to 1 teaspoon diluted, twice a day in the morning and evening. This formula can be expected to bring some improvement in a few days, but more certain results take one to two weeks. It can be taken safely for up to three weeks, by which time reassessment by a care provider is recommended. Some infections are notoriously hard to clear once and for all. If any infection is still present but seems to be responding to the herbs, another three weeks and a retest are wise. In chronic states of infection requiring more than six weeks of herbal therapy, double-check dietary and other recommendations to make sure the cause has been identified and is being handled. If it is, these herbs can be used over the long term by skipping one day each week, for up to six months.

Eight ounces will last about two weeks, the length of time for herbs to support the immune system's return to health and elimination of infection.

Sometimes, if bacteria are allowed to thrive in a dry or overdouched vaginal environment, they may cause a bladder infection (cystitis) and ascending kidney infection. Though these conditions require diagnosis by a physician, herbs and other natural treatments can help eliminate them. A woman with a kidney infection should not try to self-treat with herbs unless she is experienced with treating this naturally. Older women with a urinary tract infection (UTI) can develop dangerous conditions, so if there is a UTI and any fever, get it checked out. When the first warning signs of a bladder infection come on (difficulty in urinating or pain on passing urine), prevent their progression by drinking more plain water than usual every day. Cranberry juice can also help: every two hours for two to four days, as needed, drink an 8-ounce glass of juice to which has been added a pinch of baking soda (not baking powder).

If the water or cranberry juice isn't helping, try the following herbal tea. Herbal teas work better for bladder infections than concentrated extracts or capsules because the water helps flush out invading organisms from the kidneys and bladder without too much extra effort. You will need to visit the bathroom frequently during this cleansing process.

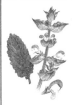

Tea for the urinary tract

DRIED HERBS	ACTIONS
2 oz. bearberry leaf (*Arctostaphylos uva-ursi*)	Helps disinfect urinary tract
1 oz. echinacea root (*Echinacea purpurea*)	Fights microorganisms directly; increases natural resistance
1 oz. cramp bark (*Viburnum opulus*)	Reduces painful urination, spasms
2 oz. linden flower (*Tilia* species)	Relaxes nerves; for circulation and taste
2 oz. parsley leaf (*Petroselinum crispum*)	Helps kidneys flush out urine

Add ½ ounce of the mixture to 3 cups of boiling water in a teapot or container with a well-fitting lid. Let stand for fifteen minutes and then strain. Drink 1 cup, hot or cold, every two hours for the first three days, then reduce tea to 1 cup three times a day. It may not take all fourteen days to feel better, but finish up the tea whether or not you have symptoms—your bladder and immune system will thank you. After these two weeks, your kidneys will have been supported so well that your skin may feel smoother, a bonus for not stopping the tea too soon. If you substitute fresh organic parsley for dried, use one standard organic grocery-store bunch (about a large handful) every three days (one-third bunch per day). Commercial parsley is loaded with pesticides that you do not want in your teacup.

Eight ounces will last two weeks.

Note: If a repeated or severe infection accompanied by fever or other signs does not respond well to herbs in two or three days, contact a qualified health-care provider.

Nutrition

Review the following suggestions for whole foods that provide vitamins and minerals to address vaginal problems, as well as the list of natural supplements.

wise food choices

❀ Use garlic, a source of zinc and other relevant nutrients.

❀ The wide variety of whole foods that are rich in phytosterols help alleviate vaginal atrophy. These include beans and legumes, sprouted seeds, nuts, pomegranates, dates, carrots, yams, real licorice candy, and real ale (made with hops).

❀ Avoid sugar and refined and processed foods. Even honey, maple syrup, and an excess of sweet fruit juices may interfere with the body's ability to fight infection, especially when vaginitis is associated with chronic yeast.

❀ Eat sour fruits (lemon, grapefruit, cranberries, plums) in season. Drink one glass daily of cranberry juice; use the bottled type that is naturally sweetened with white grape juice and dilute with an equal part of pure water; avoid brands containing glucose and corn syrup.

supplements

❀ Vitamin E can help with vaginal problems, especially thinning and dryness. In a study of forty-seven women who were taking 500 I.U. of vitamin E per day, two-thirds were helped; half of this group who had vaginal lesions due to thinning or drying were healed.

❀ Zinc helps heal inflammation and tears in the vaginal wall, and it's useful for other wounds, too.

In Addition

❀ You can participate in intercourse as long as you do not have an infection and it feels enjoyable. Sex stimulates secretion of mucus from the vaginal walls.

❀ Practice pelvic floor exercises for five minutes a day. See page 31.

❀ Natural lubricants can make a big difference. These are not simply herbal versions of petroleum jelly. Licorice, calendula, St. John's wort, and comfrey heal minor tears, soften and moisten, fight infection, and lessen inflammation. Wild yam oil is the basis for many natural creams used specifically in menopause for improving vaginal lubrication. The herb's plant sterols (phytosterols) have a beneficial effect on the vagina and a woman's entire system, but there is no certainty that wild yam or other herbal preparations with phytosterols for vaginal or skin massage increase estrogen. They do have remarkable anti-inflammatory and healing properties, regardless of the exact biochemical mechanism. Many natural lubricants are available for sale in herb shops and natural-food stores and from mail-order businesses; see Resources.

❋ You may want to make an all-natural herbal salve; see "Nourishing Herbal Salve for Vaginal Comfort" on page 32 and ready-made products in the Resources section. Making your own salve is a great way to incorporate herbs into your daily life. At first it may be messy, but it is always fun and smells terrific.

❋ A still easier way to combine healing herbs for your vagina is to add essential oils from plants (not blends or perfumes of flowers) to liquid vitamin E oil. See "Sexuality and Vaginal Changes" on page 27.

❋ The following is a soothing vaginal application for inflammation that does not dry the tissues. Boil ¼ cup water to sterilize, then cool to a comfortably cool temperature. Add 2 tablespoons aloe vera gel and whisk or stir briskly until the gel is mixed well into the water. There will still be some clumps. Use 1 to 2 tablespoons at a time; cover and refrigerate the rest. Wash your hands well, then spread the labia apart with one hand, and apply the mixture with the other. Insert a few fingerfuls into the canal without forcing. Gently massage it into the vaginal opening and outer labia, wherever extra soothing is needed. Wash hands well again; wear old underwear or relax where you can wear none at all for an hour or two. Repeat twice daily for up to a week, then repeat every once in a while as needed. This mixture works well when used over a few months, alternating as desired with the vaginal salve described on page 32.

❋ Some practitioners recommend that women never douche, but in my experience, rinsing out the lower vaginal canal and gently cleansing the labia helps the body's natural defenses resolve simple infections. Follow directions that come with every store-bought douche bag. The applicator is inserted as shallowly as possible, not high up in the vaginal canal. This formula is *for external use only*. Combining vulnerary (wound-healing) teas and an antimicrobial essential oil, it helps with vaginal infections caused by menopausal changes rather than simply rehydrating dry or thin vaginal membranes. It may seem silly to say "external use only" when we all know the vagina is an inner passage, but it means that the mixture is not to be taken by *mouth* because it includes a strong essential oil.

❋ Yogurt is an old standby of kitchen medicine that sometimes works but is mainly effective for minor yeast infections. Use plain, live culture, organic yogurt (not the flavored kind with fruit at the bottom). Apply a teaspoon at a time, liberally swabbing it on reddened, sore spots with clean fingers. Wear a panty liner, flannel menstrual pad, or old underwear. The yogurt stays in most effectively while you lie horizontally (ideally, during your overnight sleep time).

❋ Goldenseal (*Hydrastis canadensis*) is a popular herbal remedy but it is now endangered in the wild from overharvesting. Herbalists prefer now to replace it with Oregon mountain grape root (*Mahonia aquifolium*, also sold as *Berberis aquifolium*) or yerba mansa root (*Anemopsis californica*), whichever is available in your region or from reputable herb suppliers (see Resources). Use 1 ounce of powdered herb to 1 pint of water as a vaginal douche every day for three days. If the infection is not completely cleared up, or if there is fever and worsening symptoms at any time, see your health-care professional.

❋ Meditation and visualization can bring profound healing to the physical body by uniting it with the nonphysical aspects of ourselves. See page 86 for one suggested meditation.

Herbal douche for vaginal infections

5 oz. yarrow flower *(Achillea millefolium)*

5 oz. calendula flower *(Calendula officinalis)*

4 drops essential oil of marjoram per cup of tea (directions follow)

Combine the yarrow and calendula flowers. Ten ounces will last ten days. To make the douche solution, add 1 ounce of the two-herb mixture to 2 cups of boiling water, cover, and steep for forty-five minutes or until cool to the touch. Do not add the essential oil while the tea is still hot or it will evaporate and be less effective. After the tea is cool to the touch, strain, then add four drops of essential oil to 6 to 8 ounces of the strong herb tea. The marjoram oil works best when dispersed thoroughly in the herb tea, so stir, whisk, or shake well. Pour into a sterilized douche bag, available from drugstores and supermarkets in the pharmacy section.

Sitting on a toilet, lean back, and insert the applicator about an inch or two into the vaginal canal (there's no need to go deeper). Holding the bag up and squeezing gently, let the herbal liquid flow in. It isn't necessary to hold the herbal liquid in; let it flow out of the vagina and into the toilet bowl. You don't have to rinse afterward, because the herbs have an anti-inflammatory, antimicrobial, and astringent action on the vaginal walls—not drying, but toning and moistening. Sterilize the douche bag and applicator with a mild antiseptic and boiling water after every use. Dry the equipment before storing it. Repeat application once or twice daily, depending on the infection's severity and the duration of relief. Continue for no more than ten days. Whether or not antibiotics or other medication are needed, you can safely use this douche in combination with the herbal tea described previously, to support the urinary tract.

Meditation for Emotional Balance

Have someone read this to you, or record yourself reading it and play it back. If you record it, you may wish to leave a silent pause of twenty-five seconds or more where asterisks (*) appear. The entire meditation can last as briefly as three minutes or as long as an hour—it's up to you and the time you have available. Sit or lie comfortably and close your eyes for the meditation.

Breathe deeply. Relax any tension you may feel in your jaw or neck. *

Put aside any thoughts you may have for just this moment; allow your inner eye to gaze on a landscape of symbols—geometric shapes, meanings expressed in color, or pictures that are not logical yet are true for you. Because this journey is in your imagination, you can stop at any time, undisturbed, still in charge of your Self. Breathe in deeply and breathe out slowly.

In your mind's eye, take all your attention to the center of your body—the very center. It is about halfway down your body, about four inches below your navel. There, almost invisible because it is not truly physical, a seed of pure energy vibrates. This seed crystal of your essence vibrates with every color of the light spectrum, flashing red, then the orange of a harvest moon, solar yellow, garden green, sky blue, midnight blue, and celestial violet. *

In your imagination, let your inner eye see the vibration of red, so deeply red that it could be the seed from which all red grows. It is the red of the rose that can take your breath away. The rose perfumes our world with a wild and cultured love whose language is fragrance.

Breathe and relax. Let this rose red open before your inner eye into a bud of palest pink. Watch and continue to breathe evenly as it deepens to a warm pink blush, followed by the deepest burgundy of a mature bloom. *

Rich red, the vibration of blood, river of life. Now rose colors from your center diffuse through your every cell, cascading like a waterfall of burgundy rose petals, nourishing your womb, your ovaries—even if they have been removed. This wise vibration nourishes the body memory of your perfectly integrated creative center. Let it fall and rise to flow to every layer of tissue, kissing every living cell. This red flows to heal any wounds you may have received; let them receive healing, forgiveness, your compassionate and full attention. *

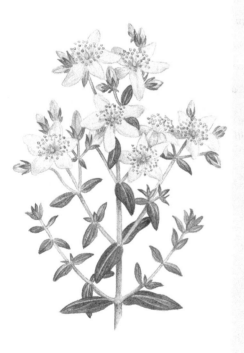

With your inner eye you may see this red glow brighten and dim, ebb and flow, as it brings wisdom. Its vibration responds to the pull of the moon, yet this rose red will not flow out of you to nourish the Earth or even to mother a new little life. It is kept inside for nourishing your being, birthing your renewed woman's spirit. When it no longer flows in rosy rivers outside of us, it flows mysteriously within our blood to nourish deep wellsprings within our Earth, our bodies, the peak of our beings. You are connected to the red center of our planetary body. Fiery energy from the timeless internal ocean of Earth's central flame rises through layers of earth to bring you living rose red, blood red, fiery red life for the work you have taken on. *

Gently bring your attention back to your whole body, and breathe evenly. When you feel ready, open your eyes.

CHANGING APPEARANCE OF SKIN AND HAIR

You'll notice that your hair and skin become drier at menopause. This change is due not solely to declining estrogen but also to shifting levels of nutrients and hormones in general. Now, more than ever, you need to eat well, optimize circulation to the skin and scalp, and protect the outer surface of your body to avoid dry skin and hair.

The herbs for strengthening bone resiliency and suggestions for preventing osteoporosis also help with hair and skin. Dry hair and skin also can be conditioned by regular use of moisturizing plants and oils. Aromatic plants with oils—for example, rosemary, sage, lemon balm, and lemon grass—make good daily hair rinses. Dry or mature skin responds well to the moisturizing herbs, especially comfrey, chamomile, sandalwood, and calendula. These are also called *vulnerary* or wound healing, because they speed the body's self-repair of scratches, burns, rashes, wounds, and other "vulnerable" places on the surface of the scalp and skin.

Women have been using herbs for hair care for millennia, including less-usual cosmetic aids such as black walnut, cloves, coffee, and henna, and extracted oils such as olive, jojoba, and vitamin E. The beauty of getting on in years is that our skin actually softens, unless we callus it with rough treatment or overexposure to chemicals and sun. An old lady's face is wonderfully soft, like a baby's. No matter what we have done with our skin and hair in the past decades, a six-month regimen of the following extract and/or tea nourishes body and soul, from the inside out.

Let us never bother to lie about our age or try to hide it. These recommendations are for vibrant health and the fun of using plants, not as a cover-up.

Herbal Medicine

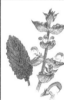

Concentrate for changes to the skin

CONCENTRATED HERB EXTRACT	ACTIONS
3 oz. plantain leaf (*Plantago major, P. minor, P. ovata, P. lanceolata*)	Moistening; helps liver balance hormones; for taste
2 oz. nettle leaf (*Urtica dioica*)	Mineralizing nutritive; tonic for good elimination
2 oz. wild yam root (*Dioscorea villosa*)	Nourishes skin; anti-inflammatory; improves lower intestinal function
1 oz. rosemary flower, leaf (*Rosmarinus officinalis*)	Optimizes circulation; aids assimilation of nutrients

Combine these herbal extracts. Take 1 teaspoon in 1 cup of water, diluted juice, or herb tea in the morning and evening.

Eight ounces will last two weeks.

Tea for changes to the skin

DRIED HERBS	ACTIONS
3 oz. lemon grass leaf (*Cymbopogon* species)	Moistening; for taste
2 oz. linden flower (*Tilia platophyllos, T. europaea*)	Nourishes skin; anti-inflammatory; relaxing nervine; mild vasodilator (lowers high blood pressure); for taste
2 oz. nettle leaf (*Urtica dioica*)	Mineralizing nutritive; tonic for good elimination
1 oz. or less, to taste, rosemary flower, leaf (*Rosmarinus officinalis*)	Optimizes circulation, assimilation of nutrients

Add ½ ounce of the mixture to 3 cups of boiling water in a teapot or container with a well-fitting lid. Let stand for fifteen minutes and then strain. If it tastes too strong, add water or reduce the rosemary. Drink 1 cup, hot or cold, one to three times a day. If you prefer, sip tea off and on throughout the day.

Eight ounces will last at least two weeks.

My favorite external herbal formula for dry hair is a combination I learned from two beautiful Moroccan herbal students. It can be used to condition or naturally tint the hair, and it's easy to create variations with each batch. The main variation for many readers may be the use or avoidance of henna powder (*Lawsonia inermis*). Henna comes in red, neutral, and other colors, and though this Egyptian cosmetic herb is useful, it takes one or two times of experimenting with the henna-powder-and-water mud pack to feel that you know what you are doing, and the results vary, naturally. A little goes a long way. Overuse of henna (every few months for two or more years) is drying to the hair, especially if it is mixed with water alone. The other herbs and oils in this combination minimize that problem, but when in doubt, leave the henna out. Enjoy!

Samia and Fatima's Diamanda Special

DRIED HERBS	ACTIONS
2 oz. rosemary leaf, flower (*Rosmarinus officinalis*)	Conditions; darkens gray
1 oz. horsetail leaves (*Equisetum arvense*)	Coats hair shaft with minerals
1 oz. chamomile flower (*Matricaria recutita*)	Volatile oils nourish, add moisture
1 oz. nettle leaf (*Urtica dioica*)	Conditions hair and scalp
½ oz. black walnut hulls (*Juglans nigra*)	Darkens; covers gray
½ oz. clove powder (*Eugenia caryophyllata*)	Volatile oils nourish, add moisture
½ oz. ground coffee (*Coffea* species)	Volatile oils nourish, add moisture
Hot water (not quite boiling) sufficient to make a paste	Keeps henna from overdrying hair
1 to 8 tbsp. olive oil	Conditions hair
Optional: 1 to 4 oz. henna powder (*Lawsonia inermis*)	Colors cover gray with neutral, red, brown, or other desired color pigments

Other items you may need: mirror, drinking water, clock, comb, glass or ceramic bowl, plastic gloves, shower cap, at least one old towel, washcloth, mild shampoo, moisturizer or facial cream

Grind the herbs to a fine powder in a blender or one at a time in a coffee grinder. Remove as many stems as you have the patience to sift out. Stir powders together. In a nonmetal covered container (glass or ceramic bowl with a lid or a salad bowl and a plate), pour the hot water over the herbs and soak, covered, for ten minutes.

continued on page 90

Position the mirror, drinking water, clock, comb, bowl, plastic gloves, and at least one old towel near the sink. Cover the surrounding floor (an old shower curtain makes a good floor covering). Lightly shampoo hair; towel dry. Place a thin line of moisturizer or facial cream around the hairline, including the tops of your ears, to avoid staining facial skin. Stir the oil into the wet herb mixture to create a smooth paste of oatmeal consistency. The mixture should neither run through the fingers nor crumble into dry lumps. Add spoonfuls of water or oil to get the right consistency. If it gets too wet, add more powdered dry herbs.

Divide your clean, damp hair into sections and apply this herb goo, massaging it into the scalp. It may make a mess, so go slowly and have fun. Use a damp washcloth frequently to wipe any drips from your neck and face. When hair is covered with an even thickness, roots to ends, swish a few spoonfuls of warm water in the henna bowl to make a little herb-flecked "tea" to pat on or pour over the mud pack on your head. This ensures that the mixture soaks down evenly to the roots of your hair.

Cover your hair with an old towel or shower cap. The herb mixture shouldn't get dry over the next fifteen to ninety minutes, so keep your scalp wet—if necessary, by covering your hair first with a shower cap or plastic bag or by periodically changing to a new hot, wet towel. Keep drinking water or herb teas, as you may not notice that you are becoming dehydrated from the warmth. After fifteen minutes, rinse out a test strand. Don't worry—this isn't like using plain henna. Left on hair too long without these botanical helpers to soften its effects, henna can make hair too brassy and too dry. Once I fell asleep with this formula on for four hours and my hair didn't go orange, but it sure was deeply conditioned! Depending on your test strand, gauge your remaining time with a maximum of ninety minutes—the longer the time, the deeper the color and/or conditioning. After fifteen to ninety minutes, or when you have had enough, or the weight of the mud pack and towel tires your neck muscles, remove the towel and/or shower cap and get into the shower. Rinse out the herbs with plain water before using diluted mild shampoo, mixed with about half water. Then massage the shampoo into the hair and scalp with gentle motions. When fully lathered, rinse and repeat as needed. You will probably wash your hair several times; if you like, condition as usual. The first day your hair may feel dry, but from the second day on it will shine.

Repeat once every six to twelve weeks as desired but not more than four to six times a year, total. Henna is a stain, after all, and overuse can cause eventual allergic sensitivity—the irritation is your body's way of letting you know it's no longer okay to use so much. This same herb conditioning can be repeated without henna for one or two hours as often as you like.

Herbal and essential oils are used in every culture to nourish hair and skin. These plants combine anti-inflammatory properties with cleansing, antibacterial, and moisturizing effects.

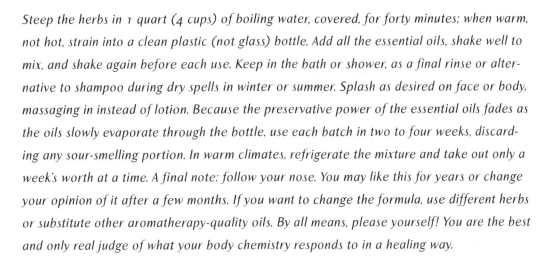

Aromatic skin and hair rinse

1 oz. comfrey leaf or root *(Symphytum officinale)*

½ oz. chamomile flower *(Matricaria recutita)*

¼ oz. calendula flower *(Calendula officinalis)*

15 drops essential oil of sandalwood *(Santalum album)*

5 drops essential oil of rosemary *(Rosmarinus officinalis)*

3 drops essential oil of lemon grass *(Cymbopogon citratus)*

Steep the herbs in 1 quart (4 cups) of boiling water, covered, for forty minutes; when warm, not hot, strain into a clean plastic (not glass) bottle. Add all the essential oils, shake well to mix, and shake again before each use. Keep in the bath or shower, as a final rinse or alternative to shampoo during dry spells in winter or summer. Splash as desired on face or body, massaging in instead of lotion. Because the preservative power of the essential oils fades as the oils slowly evaporate through the bottle, use each batch in two to four weeks, discarding any sour-smelling portion. In warm climates, refrigerate the mixture and take out only a week's worth at a time. A final note: follow your nose. You may like this for years or change your opinion of it after a few months. If you want to change the formula, use different herbs or substitute other aromatherapy-quality oils. By all means, please yourself! You are the best and only real judge of what your body chemistry responds to in a healing way.

Nutrition

Review the following suggestions for whole foods that provide vitamins and minerals to address skin and hair issues, as well as the list of natural supplements.

wise food choices

- ❀ Eat soy foods, unless you are allergic to them.

- ❀ Drink 1 teaspoon of freshly ground flaxseed meal stirred into a glass of water once a day for at least two months.

- ❀ Eat a quarter or half avocado twice a week in salads or garlic vegetable dip (guacamole is great, but not with bags of tortilla chips). Spread avocado on whole-grain toast.

* Eat one or two pieces of organic seasonal fruit per day, followed with water or herb tea.

* For better blood sugar, appetite control, energy levels, and metabolism, eat fruit with 1 teaspoon raw sunflower seeds or five to ten raw, unsalted almonds. Chew slowly.

* Avoid all heated, hydrogenated, or partially hydrogenated oils and fats (margarine, commercial bakery items).

* Avoid refined sugars.

supplements

* Omega-3 capsules, as directed on label

* Evening primrose oil, three capsules three times a day for one to six months

In Addition

* Women in their fifties may feel ultrasensitive about how they are perceived. Your looks do not "go," but they do change. Turn your back on powerful media messages aimed at your vanity and your purse. A truly feminine spirit at this time of life is more similar to that of a mature tigress—who can be serenely contented or powerfully pissed off—than to a sappy TV mannequin.

* Define beauty for yourself. White, silver, or gray hair is beautiful. Set it with silver hair combs and get it conditioned, braided, or cut in a new way you've always wanted to see on yourself.

* Make an aromatic rinse for your skin and hair (see page 91).

* Exercise, exercise, exercise! It sweats out impurities, decreases tension, optimizes circulation, and releases hormones for immune health and an uplifted mood.

* Take saunas as often as you wish or can tolerate.

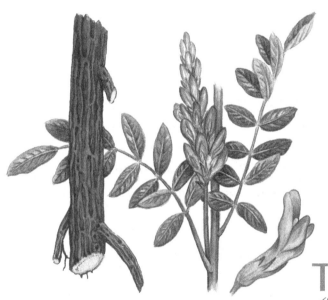

chapter 3
Hormone Replacement Therapy

The idea behind hormone replacement therapy (HRT) and estrogen replacement therapy (ERT)– that all symptoms of menopause can be reversed or avoided with hormone supplements–makes sense only if you believe that menopause is simply a deficiency of estrogen. To review, the physical symptoms of menopause include: hot flashes, night sweats, vaginal dryness, bladder control problems, insomnia/disrupted sleep, palpitations, dryness and thinning of the skin, headaches, weight gain, breast tenderness, gastrointestinal distress and nausea, tingling or itchy skin, buzzing in the head, electric shock sensation, bloating, sore joints/muscles, hair loss or thinning, increase in facial hair, changes in body odor, dry mouth, and other oral symptoms. The emotional signs of menopause include: irritability, mood swings, depression, lowered libido, anxiety, brain fog (difficulty concentrating and confusion), memory lapses, extreme fatigue/low energy levels, and feeling emotionally detached. This list of symptoms is very diverse, from small discomforts to major problems. Estrogen alone is not the solution, nor is progesterone alone. Despite their general acceptance by the American medical profession in past decades, however, Hormone Replacement Therapy (HRT), Hormone Therapy (HT), and Estrogen Replacement Therapy (ERT) are not really therapies at all, but drug treatments. Therapy implies that treatment will result in a cure. Drug treatment overlaps with this definition but does not necessarily mean there is ever an end of the need for drugs: powerful, concentrated hormones taken throughout and after the menopausal transition. This chapter discusses the pros and cons of taking hormones and "natural" sources of hormones. Bioidentical hormones (bHRT) have been a successful option for many (well-publicized) women. But practitioners find that women feel their best when their treatment is customized to them personally because there are different forms of bioidentical HRT that work in different ways. Also in this chapter are herbal remedies that you can safely take along with HRT and that help you slowly come off of it. You might ask, do I need to wean off of HRT? Current data suggests strongly that the best results for women taking hormones are in the first three years of perimenopause. After that, the risks outweigh the benefits.

HRT STUDIES: THE PROS AND CONS OF THE DRUGS

When considering whether to use a drug we always want to look at the studies done to determine its efficacy (that is, how well it works for what we are trying to treat) and its safety. There are many problems in examining studies. Most important is that no two women are the same. Variables not always reflected in studies include dietary practices (vegetarian, low-fat, meat-eating, fiber content, and so forth), body weight, liver function, types of intestinal bacteria, time between eating and eliminating (transit time), hormonal enzyme activity, and age—all factors that can influence hormone production and utilization, as well as overall health. The several kinds of estrogen that are made naturally in the body or that are converted through metabolism make a big difference, too. One problem in identifying the risks and benefits of taking hormones is that studies look at narrow questions and answers such as those differences between women's choices and risk factors throughout life. When looking at the results of studies we then have to apply the information to individual women. We also have to remember that studies are not the gospel truth, whether we agree or disagree with the results. All are worth consideration; few are worth banking on.

Advantages of HRT

According to reviews of medical literature by the National Women's Health Network (www .womenshealthnetwork.org), HRT may be a wise choice in menopause for (1) relieving the symptoms of extreme hot flashes, (2) helping insomnia caused by night sweats, (3) lessening risk of severe osteoporosis, and (4) preventing extreme vaginal dryness. The U.S. Food and Drug Administration (FDA) has approved it only for preventing osteoporosis. In my opinion, I find the outlook of the national women's health group most helpful. In their view, HRT is useful only when (1) natural methods have not been able to alleviate the problems a woman is having, (2) she understands that HRT will suppress her symptoms, not "cure" her, (3) she knows the risks of taking hormones and can accept those risks, (4) the prescription improves her quality of life, and (5) the benefits outweigh the risks—in a woman with multiple risk factors for severe osteoporosis. Drugs are not "bad" compared with all-natural herbs; a woman's well-being is more important than moral judgments about whether it came from natural approaches or synthetic sources.

Disadvantages of HRT

The disadvantages of HRT are many. Women who are not candidates for taking hormones include those who have high blood pressure, uterine fibroids, diabetes, estrogen-dependent breast cancer now or in the past, any significant liver or gallbladder disease, or cardiovascular disease; nor should any woman use them during pregnancy.

To continue their menstrual cycles, women are usually prescribed Premarin (estrogen) (0.625 milligram every day for days one to twenty-five of the cycle), followed by Provera (progestin) (2.5, 5, or even 10 milligrams for days thirteen to twenty-five). Though the higher dosages are now reserved mainly for women under age fifty-five, there are cases of women reaching seventy-five who still have a period every month because they are on prescribed hormones such as Premarin. These women may be taking too high a dose, prescribed years earlier and never reassessed. They should not be bleeding at this age and their doses should be modulated if they are taking HRT, for example, for osteoporosis. Commonly, but not always, women over age fifty-five are switched to a continuous cycle of Premarin (0.625 milligram every day) and Provera (2.5 milligrams every day), so their periods do not continue, although estrogen-dependent fibroids, benign or other breast lumps, and menstrual migraines remain actively stimulated by the hormones. These conditions, as well as mood swings, may even worsen. The most popular estrogen used in HRT (Premarin) comes from pregnant mare's urine; other types may be totally synthetic. How this urine is "farmed" raises ethical questions. For more information, see www.hsus.org/horses_equines/issues/the_facts_ about_premarin.html.

Synthetic hormones have historically proven to have serious adverse effects associated with them. DES (diethylstilbestrol), a hormonal drug used in the late 1930s to the early 1970s for easing morning sickness in pregnant women, was found to cause breast and uterine cancer and birth defects in developing female and male offspring. However, the risks associated with its use weren't recognized until more than twenty years after it began to be prescribed, despite large numbers of prescriptions to women.

HRT may ease signs and symptoms, but high costs in health are likely over time. It has been used for several decades now and while there are certainly risks, the adverse effects are not likely to be as extreme as those of DES. Estrogen that we make in our own bodies even after menopause protects our hearts and bones, but HRT is no longer considered cardioprotective. HRT does apparently lower the risk of osteoporosis but, just like the Pill, it also increases the risk of high blood pressure, emboli that can lead to strokes, and cancer.

It is not only replacing estrogen that causes problems in menopausal women. In an early Australian review of several studies on the psychological effects of synthetic progesterone (progestin) added to estrogen in menopausal medication, the reviewers note that 85 percent of the women in one study asked to be taken off the study and the medication because of side effects; these included withdrawal bleeding that was worse than their former menstrual flows and out-of-control mood swings. Progesterones added to estrogens generate PMS-like symptoms, including simultaneous depression and agitation. Some doctors, such as John R. Lee, MD, find progesterone more helpful than estrogen for menopausal issues, and others use bioidentical hormones for improving bone density, reducing hot flashes, and optimizing other aspects of health during and after menopause. The standard approach is not all that standardized at this time. One of many reasons that naturopathic doctors and conventional medical doctors have different opinions on how to give women hormones is that new research is always replacing outdated findings. As long ago as 1989, a Consensus Conference determined that the use of progestin resulted in an increased risk of heart disease.

Even for women with surgical or medically caused menopause, natural remedies may provide ample support with fewer long-term risks. Breast cancer rates are falling as women abandon HRT, according to Cancer Research UK. The number of women under sixty taking HRT has been halved between 2000 and 2009. In February 2009, the *European Journal of Cancer* published a report that in 2000, 40 percent of women between the ages of fifty and fifty-four were on HRT. By 2006, only 20 percent of women aged fifty to fifty-four were still receiving prescribed HRT, and among fifty-five- to fifty-nine-year-olds, the percentage had dropped to fifteen.

Research on alternatives to HRT has been mixed. Six women in various medical disciplines reviewed seventy clinical trials in 2009 and concluded that "…although individual trials suggest benefits from certain therapies, data are insufficient to support the effectiveness of any complementary and alternative therapy in this review for the management of menopausal symptoms. Many of these potential therapies warrant further study in trials with rigorous scientific designs to determine benefit and safety" (Nedrow et al).

HORMONE THERAPY: A HISTORICAL OVERVIEW

When and how did ERT and HRT become the standard drug approaches to menopause? In the late 1960s, supported by a male-dominated medical system and misconceptions about women's physiologic processes, estrogen was touted as a "wonder drug," exploiting women's fears about aging, which included losing our socially accepted role as a potentially reproductive girlfriend, wife, and mother or the "alternative" role of the ever-sexy femme fatale. To judge from popular media, the dominant cultural bias still accepts the stereotype of menopausal women as neurotic, whiny, asexual, and unattractive. If a woman has laugh lines around her eyes or is no longer willing to put up or shut up, she is fit only, according to "modern" Western culture, to be put out to pasture. Older women are being medicated for being their own age. Advertisements for menopausal products in medical and popular journals frequently depict women who do not use HRT as decrepit and gray; women who use it are air-brushed, pink-lipped, and kissed by men. Meanwhile, silver-haired men with paunches are dashing around with women the age of their daughters—and their midlife crises are still applauded even as our dominant culture jokes about it. The decline of testosterone that takes place between ages forty and sixty has not been pinpointed for treatment like a woman's end of monthly cycles has been, but both transitions are real. Although many women and men today are admirably redefining social roles, the thrust of our Western culture gives only lip service to older women's rights, and that's not good enough.

By the time estrogen became one of the top five drugs prescribed in the United States in the mid-1970s, rates of uterine, ovarian, and breast cancer had increased five to fourteen times higher than previous levels, and the incidences of uterine fibroids, fibrocystic breast lumps, and gallbladder disease were far higher. These are related to HRT use in that generation of menopausal women. Gallbladder disease especially affects Native American women and women with high cholesterol, as well as women who are twenty pounds or more overweight, because body fat creates more estrogen.

When a link between the use of estrogen and cancers of the ovaries, uterus, and breasts was cautiously "suggested," prescriptions plummeted. Pharmaceutical companies had increased production, but their warehouses stayed full. Public relations firms and women doctors hired by the companies flooded television and women's magazines with carefully worded ads and new items claiming that the risks were exaggerated. Then women's health groups and a small group of concerned physicians worked with the FDA to demand warning labels on estrogen prescriptions. In 1979 the National Institutes of Health rejected the drug manufacturers' then-current marketing claims, especially as they related to HRT's psychological and physical benefits. The NIH accepted the use of HRT only for hot flashes and vaginal dryness. In the end, drug companies shifted to using combined HRT rather than ERT for women with reproductive organs, to decrease the risk of uterine cancer. However, the combination of estrogen and progesterone can result in unpleasant withdrawal bleeding and incomplete uterine shedding. Retaining tissue that is not completely shed through menstrual flow is another risk for gynecological disease.

Medical views of menopause and disease as we age are colored, from decade to decade, by cultural and philosophical views that are not as concrete as Western biomedicine wants to admit. As the Dutch professor of philosophy, Louise Derksen, has pointed out, a shift in cultural views was reflected in a 2005 *Time* magazine article on midlife and menopause:

> "This article is a reflection of the menopausal fashion of the moment—it is not a disease and present-day women are strong, vital, and emancipated, meaning that they are capable of dealing in an empowered way with the symptoms. *Time* describes midlife as a 'stressful, pivotal moment' in the lives of women. Yet the focus of the article is the idea that such a moment can be used by women to 'reinvent themselves.' The profiled women said life only got better after midlife. They were freed from the demands of reproduction and the family. They took the opportunity to make new choices in their lives and develop new careers. *Time* states, 'Women get to wrestle with their hormones through a Change of Life; but however disruptive menopause may be for some women, the changes that matter most are often more psychic and spiritual than physical. . . . They may first turn inward, ask cosmic questions, or retrieve some passion they put aside to make room for a career and family and adult responsibilities. Take a trip. Write a novel. Go back to school. Learn to kiteboard. But then, having done something to help themselves, they have a powerful urge to help others. Best of all is when they can do both at once.'"

HORMONES, HERBS, AND CANCER RISK

There are some common misconceptions about herbal sources of hormones. Fact: Herbs are not a source of bioavailable hormones for humans. Estrogen, progesterone, and DHEA (dihydroepiandrosterone) are not found in herbs, except in tiny amounts or in fundamentally different vegetable versions. (DHEA is a steroidal hormone from the adrenal glands, like cortisol, that has broad-ranging effects on health, probably including prevention of osteoporosis.) Some manufacturers claim that wild yam, for instance, is converted into the hormones a menopausal woman needs, but there is no evidence that it can be synthesized into natural hormones in the body. Wild yam is a time-honored anti-inflammatory digestive remedy, but is not a raw source of human hormone replacements. Plants do contain plant hormones (phytoestrogens, phytosterols, and others) with hormonal-type effects in the plant. Some of these may have hormonelike effects in the human body because they can bind to human cell receptors and stimulate mild hormonal actions. We know something about these effects in women because for thousands of years women have been using the plants or whole-plant extracts with fairly predictable effects—mostly as part of a plant-based diet, but also medicinally. The synthesized hormones made from raw material in herbs, such as the DHEA made from diosgenin (extracted from wild yam), have a similar structure but a different effect in the body than the botanical and food sources of phytoestrogens we consume in their natural state. "Natural progesterone" made from wild yam or other herb extracts is a pharmaceutically manipulated hormone used for its druglike effects. Products that include it may help women with symptoms, but it is misleading to call them "natural." They are not. Wild yam as a whole herb extract has anti-inflammatory sterols, and may have a mild estrogen-like effect, not progesteronal.

The difference between vegetable, animal, and synthetic hormones is as simple as the difference between eggs and egg substitutes. (If you are not interested in biochemistry, feel free to skip this section.)

Biochemically speaking, human sex steroids (sex hormones) are of three kinds: *pregnanes*, which provide the basic compound for making all kinds of progestins and corticoids; *androstanes*, for making androgens (hormones associated with masculine secondary sex characteristics in both sexes); and *estranes*, which the body can make into all types of estrogen. All three types of sex steroids have the same basic "building block," with different numbers of carbon molecules in slightly different arrangements. Minor chemical differences translate into huge sexual differences in humans. We can find some compounds in plants that are related to human sex steroids. All plants contain hormones for the plant's growth and reproduction. These are not identical to human hormones, but there is some related activity. Sterol glycosides are one example of plant hormones. The group found in ginseng (*Panax ginseng*) are called "ginsenosides." The ginsenosides can have a stimulating effect on our hormones. Sometimes this stimulation is good in menopause; sometimes it worsens health conditions. This is why herbalists always repeat ad nauseam that we have to see each woman rather than prescribe an herb for a condition. Within the limits of a book of this kind, there are several herb formulas for women to choose from if there is no herbalist nearby.

Triterpenoid saponins are a second example of herbal hormones that have an influence on our hormone balance and health—for example, the compound glycyrrhizin found in licorice root (*Glycyrrhiza glabra*). The whole plant taken medicinally is weakly estrogen-like in its effect and has other hormonal effects (anti-inflammatory) in formulas. A third type of herbal hormonal compound that has become familiar to many menopausal women today is the steroidal saponin, such as diosgenin from wild yam (*Dioscorea villosa*). It is anti-inflammatory and may have a beneficial influence on the production of hormones mentioned above. Traditional herbal practice can predict low toxicity with all these whole plants, because less important chemicals buffer or moderate the hormonal stimulation, reducing the likelihood of side effects. An isolated chemical from the plants that is manufactured into a drug is predictably less safe.

Essential oils are another type of plant compound biochemically related to sex hormones. These are often isolated (from the plant's fiber or chlorophyll, for instance) but are used in very small amounts. Their strong effects on balancing hormones have been known for much longer than pharmaceutical or synthetic hormone derivatives. This is partly because essential oils share a fundamental property bridging plant and animal life processes: cholesterol. Naturally occurring cholesterol is a basic building block for hormones in mammals. Cholesterol also forms essential oils in certain plants, though it isn't cholesterol by the time it is part of a plant. As modern food labeling keeps reminding us, plant oils are by definition cholesterol-free. The aromas of these herbs or their essential oils affect mammals powerfully. In therapeutic herbal medicine, traditional use of essential oils in context usually stimulates better internal regulation of sex hormones. This is not the same as simply stimulating an increase of sex hormones. An example of a hormone-balancing essential oil is clary sage (*Salvia sclarea*).

It makes sense that vegetables do not normally contain the same sex hormones for flowering and dropping seed that animals need for their reproduction. On the other hand, a few known plants can yield a variation that is amazingly close. The date palm (*Phoenix dactylifera*)—associated since ancient times with fertility in camels, women, and other mammals—contains a small quantity of estrone, especially during that desert tree's natural reproductive season. But other than examples such as this one, phytoestrogens fall into the two main groups identified so far. I've already talked about three categories in the first main group: the steroidal glycosides, triterpenoid saponins, and steroidal saponins found in herbs such as ginseng, licorice, and wild yam. These compounds related to sterol and cholesterol are one main group of phytoestrogens. The second main group contains the isoflavone type of phytoestrogens. Formononetin, a common isoflavone, is found in red clover (*Trifolium pratense*) and many other herbs. The bitter herb hops (*Humulus lupulus*) contains far higher amounts of formononetin than red clover and other pea family plants. But, luckily for us, we do not usually eat hops as a main course or even as a side dish of vegetables. Nature set it up so that certain powerful herbs (like hops) are too unpleasant-tasting to eat on a regular basis, thus reducing the likelihood of problems arising.

Many women are told to stop taking estrogenic herbs because their doctors do not understand what experienced herbalists know about these herbs. Herbs with effects somewhat similar to estrogen have been shown to have paradoxical effects. These effects are due to competitive binding with various hormone receptors on our cell membranes. This can result in preferential binding of weaker estrogens so that the overall load is lower, while the liver's function helps more potent estrogens to be excreted. Traditional women's herbal remedies that have helped alleviate female problems caused by high estrogen are known to contain phytoestrogens. Continuing research suggests that these herbs do not always increase a woman's estrogen. Herbs with plant hormones do not behave like hormone drugs. Some studies suggest that phytoestrogens can decrease the risk of cancer, presumably by competing with estrogen, which can cause cancer.

Some herbal remedies for menopause contain the plant hormone beta-sitosterol, and the herbs they contain only act like estrogen in women whose estrogen is unusually low. Examples of herbs containing some amount, large or small, of beta-sitosterol are dong quai, licorice, ginseng, saw palmetto, calendula, St. John's wort, and red clover. Others containing phytoestrogens, such as alfalfa, showed both estrogenic and anti-estrogenic effects in experiments, though these animal experiments from the 1960s are, in my opinion, always suspect. Having said that, this maybe-yes-maybe-no test result is in keeping with the results for other plants that, like alfalfa, contain both isoflavones and coumestrol.

The wonderful gynecologic herb chaste berry or chaste tree (*Vitex agnus-castus*) is native to the Greek islands and sacred to the goddess Hera, mythological protectress of married women and mothers. This herb affects the pituitary gland in the brain, with effects on luteinizing hormone, follicle-stimulating hormone, and prolactin. In menopause, FSH and LH are higher. Herbalists commonly speak of chaste berry as promoting progesterone. Although it appears that way, this action is unproven. A more exact description is that chaste berry promotes the rebalancing of hormonal signals between the brain and the ovaries. In turn, this action helps optimize progesterone and estrogen levels. The actual center of control is the hypothalamus, which produces a gonadotropin releasing hormone (GnRH) that stimulates the anterior pituitary to release FSH and LH. In health, the hypothalamus secretes GnRH at a pulsed rate. This is necessary for the pituitary to release the appropriate amounts of LH and FSH. Chaste berry has been shown to affect different aspects of reproductive health. In girls past the age of puberty and women of reproductive age, chaste berry has been found in more than one clinical trial to reduce PMS, acne, breast pain, and irregularity of menses. For promoting natural fertility, chaste berry increases luteinizing hormone levels (LH), while mildly inhibiting the release of follicle stimulating hormone (FSH). This indirectly boosts progesterone production and chances of achieving and maintaining a successful pregnancy. Chaste berry decreases high levels of prolactin (PL), associated with breast pain in PMS and fertility problems. It does not appear to lower normal levels of PL. In menopause, chaste berry reduces some women's hot flashes better than the popular black cohosh, which reduces LH through competitive binding at hormone receptors, among other effects of the whole root extract. In most human studies, there is a consistent finding that taking chaste berry for a minimum of three months gives better results. This is a reflection of its gentle, indirect normalization of reproductive system hormones through the complex pathways governed by the neuroendocrine system.

Another herb (in this case, a fruit) known for its hormonal health is the pomegranate, which, like the date palm, contains some trace amounts of estrone. The pomegranate is known generally for its antioxidant power. It may be that further research will measure whether there is an appreciable effect on hormone levels, and if so, how that differs between men and women, and between women at different stages of life.

Among the herbs that contain diosgenin, sarsapogenin, or related compounds are wild yam (*Dioscorea villosa*), blue cohosh (*Caulophyllum thalictroides*), fenugreek (*Trigonella foenum-graecum*), wild sarsaparilla (*Smilax* species), and bethroot (*Trillium* species), which is now endangered by overharvesting. As we now know, the botanical compounds are not converted into the stronger hormones we mammals use. Yet each herb has an effect on reproductive health. Some require training in the use of herbs and caution, such as blue cohosh (not to be confused with black cohosh, a standard herb in Western menopausal treatments).

NATURAL HORMONE REPLACEMENT OR HRT: YOUR DECISION

As baby boomers turned to natural products for coping with aging, including herbs for menopausal concerns, physicians were not the only people jumping to false conclusions about "estrogenic" herbs. The market was flooded with herbal products providing natural progesterone that may have pronounced effects on a woman's health when used as directed. Some may be made with the best intentions of providing women with alternatives to synthetic hormones. But let's be clear: no amount of external creams or ingested herbal products from these whole plants have been shown to cause an increase in a woman's estrogen or progesterone. The whole herbs and genuinely natural products made from them have many other healing attributes for women in menopause; increasing sex hormone levels is not one of them. These herbal steroids are converted into progesterone not *naturally* in our metabolism but rather in the lab. If a company claims that a month's worth of cream containing wild yam extract (a two-ounce jar) delivers 900 milligrams of "natural progesterone," it cannot have made the cream without doctoring the herbal diosgenin in the laboratory. Some companies simply use wild yam extracts and add animal progesterone, usually from "affordable raw materials." This is the polite phrase for pregnant mare's urine—the same ingredient that drug companies make into Premarin.

There is no agreement on the optimal type of drug regime or duration of monitoring by physicians when hormones are medically indicated for a menopausal woman. It *is* agreed that HRT's side effects are in proportion to the strength of the dose and the length of time on it.

Progesterone, like estrogen, may lower the incidence of bone loss, but the route of administration and the long-term effects of HRT for this effect are still debated. Patches and creams release hormones directly into the bloodstream, so the risks of high blood levels of estrogen (emboli, high blood pressure) may apply. Vaginal creams release hormones into the bloodstream as well, but in very small amounts. If the hormones are administered orally (pills), the liver can process the hormones like any drug or substance taken by mouth. But this is associated with a two to three times higher risk of gallbladder disease. As with gallbladder problems, there is an uncertain relationship between estrogen levels and osteoporosis. Though osteoporosis is a real condition, only one-quarter of postmenopausal women develop it in the ten to twenty years *after* menopause, and even then it is linked with many factors other than low estrogen levels. As for osteoporosis tests, they have their problems as well. They are expensive and so are less likely to be done in a consistent way. They may also be misleading. One examination will measure the forearm's bone density, but this says little about a woman's weight-bearing vertebrae or hip. If another costly test measures the spine and hips, it is still unclear how much bone loss in one location leads to a risk of fracture. If there are no signs or symptoms of osteoporosis in a young to middle-aged woman, the tests for predicting it may be especially inconclusive. A CT ("cat") scan has the same drawbacks but with a higher radiation dose. If bone tests are required because of personal or family history, ask your health-care provider to suggest the best type for you.

Women who do or do not experience hot flashes can have the same circulating amount of estrogen, so taking hormones is no guarantee of avoiding hot flashes. And why should women avoid them, unless they are debilitating? The opportunity to tune into the messages of the body's wisdom means clearing symptoms rather than medicating each one separately. Moreover, symptoms recur on withdrawal from hormones, which a woman may choose to do every three to six months. This allows a woman to reassess whether natural remedies have helped her make any health progress. Further, a woman and her physician can check the need for renewing a prescription or lowering the dosage. Vaginal estrogen creams are better when used briefly, if at all. The natural approach for the symptom of vaginal thinning is often as reliable, especially for sensitive women. It involves pelvic floor exercises, love (including self-love), and sexual arousal and release, or natural lubricants with a local effect of increasing tissue levels of estrogen.

Most women find added hormones superfluous even if they have not been taking perfect care of their health. That is not to say that hormones are always superfluous. Natural therapists will honor the healing value of any approach, including HRT, if it is truly healing in the context of a woman's life. Some women are helped by HRT. We all deserve respect for our health choices, without judgment from "healers" or ourselves. Talk with other women. Don't take my word for any of this. Don't take the word of a drug representative. Or a doctor. Or an herbalist. And certainly not a manufacturer of products. Don't take the word of any *one* provider as *the* answer.

PREMATURE MENOPAUSE

Premature menopause is defined as a sudden or unhealthy drop in estrogen, after puberty but before the normal age range of menopause (thirty-six to sixty-five, with fifty-one being the average age). In some cultures the mid- to late thirties are not considered an unhealthy age for menopause. Dixie Mills, MD, writes that in Japan, natural menopause begins in the early forties. Literally translated, the term for this change, *konenki*, is composed of *ko* (renewal and regeneration), *nen* (year or years), and *ki* (season or energy). Cultural anthropology has led to rethinking our definition of early menopause as premature ovarian failure. Human biocultural adaptations of menopause, birth, and reproduction are reflections of the life cycle and growth. Adjustments to life in different environments, such as the Arctic, high altitudes, and the desert, alter onset of puberty, decline in fertility, and natural menopause. The first irregular cycles and hot flashes at this age do not automatically mean there is a health problem. There may be simple causes, remedied naturally at this stage. If self-care and use of herbs doesn't resolve a woman's symptoms in three months or so, it may help to see a health professional. The ovaries may not ovulate every month, and some hormonal changes may be felt long before menopause. It is possible that our views on the age range will evolve, with population pressure, stress effects across contemporary cultures, and the exposure of people across the planet to endodisruptors (chemicals in the environment that alter reproductive health).

Premature menopause is something else. If a woman enters menopause before she has matured into it naturally, the cause may be some form of ill health. This is often linked to smoking, chemotherapy, radiation, and, of course, surgical removal of reproductive organs at any age. Conventional medicine holds that leaving in the ovaries allows a "natural" menopause, but an estimated half of the women who have undergone removal of the uterus but not the ovaries still lose some or all ovarian function. Why do ovaries stop functioning sooner than expected when not connected to a uterus? Because women react differently to traumas, including surgery, and we are not an assembly of separately moving parts. Still, sometimes this surgical choice is a woman's best chance for health, though studies show that most hysterectomies that have been performed are not medically necessary. For further information, see http://hysterectomyinformation.blogspot.com/2009_01_18_archive.html.

If presented with advice to have a hysterectomy, find a consumer health research library and a support group, whether for fibroids, endometriosis, or other pelvic conditions. Finally, seek a second and third opinion. Many surgeries, such as oophorectomy (removal of ovaries) in DES daughters (those whose mothers were given DES during the pregnancy), are a cause of premature menopause unknown in past centuries. Now, poor health at a younger age is associated with high rates of hysterectomies and the resulting high incidence of surgically-induced menopause. According to the U.S. Center for Disease Control, more than one-third of women will have had a hysterectomy by the age of sixty. The CDC also notes that the number of cases of cancer in the female reproductive tract and in the male organs is almost identical, though the incidence of male organ removal is statistically insignificant. "We have four times the hysterectomy rate of any industrialized nation, in this country," says Ernst Bartsich, a clinical associate professor at Weill Cornell Medical College. At 600,000 hysterectomies a year, this is the most common surgery performed in the United States.

Certainly, there are health risks as we grow older, but no one body organ is the cause of our most feared, most complex health problems. Our parts are built up from DNA protein blueprints found in every cell, and that does not change the minute we are done bearing children. Our body parts are not meant to be surgically removed or drugged into obedience just because someone else says we won't be needing them now. When reproductive organs hurt, this pain may be a difficult signpost to have, but it is the body's most effective way to get our attention. We may choose surgery or medication, but these are not the only possible responses to body signals. For women who are facing a surgical recommendation, this decision can be overwhelming, confusing, and terrifying. Many women are being given bad information and limited options by their doctors. But if I were bleeding heavily, in pain, missing work, unable to function, or had a family history of uterine or ovarian cancer, I'd need help making a complex decision. Support for women to figure out when surgery is in their best interest and when it is not can be found at websites such as www.safemenopausesolutions.com and www.hystersisters.com, along with many other books and resources. When healthy, the body works at *not* producing estrogenic hormones around menopause, except in smaller amounts. We are asking for trouble when we feed women a dose of hormones to "avoid health problems." We are then forced to ask why breast cancer, unexplainable endometriosis, and gynecological disease are on the rise, despite all the advances we have seen in medicine. HRT is not the sole cause of all these ills, especially if at least half the women prescribed hormones discontinue them or never start them. Our culture's lack of consciousness in our use of technology is partly responsible.

The median age for women going through a surgical menopause is forty-one, usually because of fibroids (roughly half of these women), or premature menopause due to severe illness, such as cancer. At the time of this writing, one-third of Western women over age fifty are still undergoing hysterectomies—having their "organs of hysteria" removed. There are wildly different rates for this in the United States. The statistics show two particular differences: by regions and by ethnicity, with different rates for African American, Latina, and Native American women and Caucasian women. Fibroids are a poor reason for a hysterectomy in many cases, because more conservative options exist. Surgeons have pioneered the use of myomectomies (removing just the fibroid, not the womb). Also, fibroids often shrink at menopause when estrogen levels drop naturally. At any age, women with fibroids can change the foods that affect this condition and use reproductive tonics with astringent herbs to shrink the fibroids faster while improving their general health.

With rare exceptions, women should keep their wombs. The womb is not just for carrying a pregnancy to term. This cauldron of creative life is important all through life. If a woman's womb bothers her, she might ask herself whether there is value in listening to the subtle messages her womb may convey. Some women are happier after a hysterectomy. I would not have any woman's inner journey or physical need judged. There are no pat answers, just worthwhile questions.

Even when life-threatening, noncancerous conditions make surgical menopause a lifesaving choice, the women—particularly young ones, starting HRT between twenty-six and thirty-six—do not report good results. Women thrust prematurely into menopause can first try the relevant herbal formulas and recommendations in this book. Listen to yourself first and health-care providers second—but do keep in contact with a health professional you trust.

COMING OFF OF HORMONES SAFELY

Many women already know they want to stop taking HRT and try herbs. If you have symptoms or just feel unwell on hormones, wean off of them slowly. Several dosage combinations exist. What was standard ten years ago is considered extremely high within some medical circles today. One of the more common low doses of conjugated estrogen (for example, Premarin) prescribed is 0.3 milligram. The middle dose is 0.625 milligram and the higher dose is 1.25 milligrams per day. For estradiol (for example, Estrace), the dose ranges from 0.5 milligram up to 1.0 milligram of progestin are taken for at least seven to ten days; this is repeated for three to six months. Unless your health-care provider has some outstanding reason for keeping you at the same dose, you probably can use those three to six months to slowly reduce your dosage to a lower level. At that time, women are encouraged to wean off and reassess whether they feel better without the HRT, even if they have a little bit of rebound hot flashes.

If you need to continue longer on HRT at any dose, you can start using the following herbs at the same time. Follow this safe and slow plan over the next three to six months. It may seem as if it goes on forever. But it usually is better for our bodies to follow a consistent, predictable routine when we are making major changes. If you want to go faster than this, I cannot reach out of the pages and stop you. The deciding factor is how well you are. The first step is to take the first concentrate or tea described here for at least four weeks, along with your regular dose of HRT on the regular cycle. This allows the body to recognize and get accustomed to metabolizing the milder hormone-balancing herbs before starting to slowly wean off the hormones.

If a woman is using a patch (for example, Estraderm) instead of taking oral medication, the dose is 0.05 milligram to 0.1 milligram every three to four days. This delivery of the drug (estrogen) is through the skin. Our bodies were designed to pass everything, especially hormones, through the liver. Regardless, the same herbs can be used. Lower-dose patches can be prescribed over time, or women can achieve similar results themselves.

During the first month, take the herbs along with regular use and replacement of the patch. During the next phase, wait an extra day before replacing the patch. Each time you feel ready to withstand any rebound symptoms, add another day before replacing the patch. Stretch this out as slowly as is comfortable or manageable. You can speed up the process according to your own preference. Always see a supportive health-care provider if this brings a return of symptoms that do not feel easily managed on the herbs, or even new problems. The two of you may easily identify the problems so they can be handled simply, or additional care may be required.

Herbal Medicine

Concentrate for coming off HRT

CONCENTRATED HERB EXTRACT	ACTIONS
4 oz. black cohosh root (*Cimicifuga racemosa*)	Broad-spectrum midlife support; relaxing
2 oz. fennel seed (*Foeniculum vulgare*)	Limits bloating and gas
2 oz. red clover flower (*Trifolium pratense*)	Phytoestrogen; mild lymphatic; nerve tonic

Combine these herbal tinctures or extracts. Take 1 teaspoon in 1 cup of water twice a day, morning and evening.

Eight ounces will last thirty days.

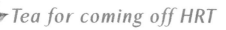

Tea for coming off HRT

DRIED HERBS	ACTIONS
2 oz. black cohosh root (*Cimicifuga racemosa*)	Broad-spectrum midlife support; relaxing
4 oz. fennel seed (*Foeniculum vulgare*)	Limits bloating and gas
2 oz. red clover flower (*Trifolium pratense*)	Phytoestrogen; mild lymphatic; nerve tonic

Add ½ ounce of the mixture to 3½ cups of boiling water in a teapot or container with a well-fitting lid. Let stand for twenty minutes before straining. Drink 1 cup, hot or cold, three times a day.

Eight ounces will last two weeks or longer.

During the second month on both the herbs and the regular HRT dose, reduce the dose of HRT by one-quarter (or less if you are very sensitive). Lowering the dose of the powerful hormones may result in a few symptoms. You can minimize symptoms by taking the second formula as concentrates (extracts) or as tea. Every time the HRT is reduced, the herb formula changes. This is usually done in one-month stages. Your body will appreciate the change of herbal flavors and benefits. You can make every stage last for two months if there is a reason to be extra cautious, such as extreme, debilitating symptoms. These combinations, when taken as directed, are safe enough for most women to take as often as they need to in order to feel well. The herbs are far more mild than the drug regime, so do not be afraid to take frequent sips of tea all day or droppers of extracts every ten minutes until you get good results.

Just for comparison, the birth control pill is 2,500 micrograms DES equivalents; postmenopausal HRT is 500 micrograms DES equivalents; and the most potent plant estrogen, coumestrol, in the form of 20 grams dry-weight soybeans (sprouted), is 0.5 microgram. This is not as weak as it looks on paper or in lab tests, because many natural plant hormones trigger activity during metabolism. Just know that vegetable hormones are not druglike in their effects.

Concentrate for smoothing the transition

EXTRACTS	ACTIONS
3 oz. peppermint leaf *(Mentha piperita)*	Reduces bloating and gas
½ oz. motherwort herb *(Leonurus cardiaca)*	Reduces hot flashes and heart palpitations
½ oz. licorice root *(Glycyrrhiza glabra)*	Anti-inflammatory; adrenal and antiviral digestive aid
1½ oz. dandelion root *(Taraxacum officinale)*	Aids liver metabolism
1½ oz. dandelion leaf *(Taraxacum officinale)*	Improves kidney function; diuretic; natural source of potassium

Combine these herbal extracts. Take 1 teaspoon in 1 cup of water twice a day, morning and evening. Women with high blood pressure or a tendency to retain water may replace the licorice with an equal amount of fennel seed, or to taste.

Seven ounces will last three weeks or longer.

Tea for smoothing the transition

DRIED HERBS	ACTIONS
1 oz. licorice root *(Glycyrrhiza glabra)*	Anti-inflammatory; adrenal and antiviral digestive aid
3 oz. peppermint leaf *(Mentha piperita)*	Reduces bloating and gas
1 oz. motherwort herb *(Leonurus cardiaca)*	Reduces hot flashes; aids liver metabolism
1½ oz. dandelion root *(Taraxacum officinale)*	Aids liver metabolism
1½ oz. dandelion leaf *(Taraxacum officinale)*	Improves kidney function; diuretic; natural source of potassium

Add ½ ounce of the mixture to 3½ cups of boiling water in a teapot or container with a well-fitting lid. Let stand for fifteen minutes before straining. Drink 1 cup, at room temperature or cold, three times a day. If you prefer, sip tea throughout the day or drink two larger glasses twice a day, but make sure you drink 3 cups a day.

Eight ounces will last two weeks or longer.

In the third month, if all is going well and you want to continue the process, reduce hormones by another one-quarter (to one-half the original dose). If you experience severe symptoms, go back to the last hormone dose that was comfortable and continue the herbs for an extra month or more, until you feel ready to try reducing the dose again. If you are very sensitive, reduce by only one-quarter at this stage, to three-quarters of the normal dose. During this month, take the following, most gentle formula for easing the transition.

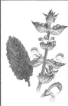

Concentrate for tapering off hormones

CONCENTRATED HERB EXTRACT	ACTIONS
2 oz. chaste berry seed (*Vitex agnus-castus*)	Promotes progesterone production through hypothalamic pathways; may reduce hot flashes
1 oz. Jamaican sarsaparilla root (*Smilax ornata*)	Hormonal balancing; lymphatic and immune tonic
2 oz. dandelion root (*Taraxacum officinale*)	Provides minerals; aids liver metabolism
2 oz. hawthorn berry (*Crataegus oxyacantha, C.* species)	Cardioprotective

Combine these herbal extracts. Take 1 teaspoon in 1 cup of water, diluted juice, or herb tea twice a day, once in the morning and once in the evening.

Seven ounces will last three weeks.

Tea for tapering off hormones

DRIED HERBS	ACTIONS
3 oz. chaste berry seed (*Vitex agnus-castus*)	Promotes progesterone; reduces hot flashes
2 oz. Jamaican sarsaparilla root (*Smilax ornata*)	Hormonal balancing; lymphatic and immune tonic
1½ oz. dandelion root (*Taraxacum officinale*)	Provides minerals; aids liver metabolism
1½ oz. hawthorn berry, leaf, and flower (*Crataegus* species) (equal parts by weight, if available)	Cardioprotective

Add ½ ounce of the mixture to 3½ cups of boiling water in a teapot or container with a well-fitting lid. Let stand for fifteen minutes before straining. Drink 1 cup, hot or cold, three times a day.

Eight ounces will last two weeks or longer.

During the fourth month, drop from one-half dose down to one-quarter dose. Once you are on a quarter dose or less, the process goes a little faster. If you are sensitive or like to take the slower method just in case, take a fifth month to drop another one-eighth off the dose. If you need to take a sixth month until you are taking one-eighth of your original dose, stay on this last herb formula, in tea or as concentrated extracts.

You may at any time go back up to the last dose of HRT and herbs that felt comfortable through the month. If this occurs more than once, pay attention to your nutrition; make sure you have outlets for stress, such as exercise, and consider other factors. Give yourself time. And let your health-care provider know what you are doing.

You will know you are ready for another dose reduction when you can honestly feel that your health signs are stable as the drugs are slowly withdrawn. Then, take only the same small dose (one-quarter or one-eighth for the very sensitive) once a week for another cycle. When you are taking the hormones only once a week, try dropping them altogether. Stay on the herb combination you are taking at that time.

The whole process of weaning off may be complete in one month or ten, but normally it will not take longer than a full year. If it does, because of other medication or chronic health issues, you may require more time or more guidance from your health-care provider.

Expecting miracles is a two-sided coin. You may have quick, terrific results, or you may feel disappointed if your symptoms are still hanging around. Herbs may or may not make your biggest symptoms disappear overnight like magic. Share your experiences with other women, but try to avoid comparing yourself with them. Look instead for longer periods of time without bad hot flashes, a few better nights of sleep in a week, or other markers you may notice.

Remember, the body in health likes rhythm. You may choose to drop your dosage at a faster rate if you have a supportive health-care provider, but whatever you do, be consistent. Quick drops in estrogen cause drops in calcium mineralization of the bone—the biggest reason for making yours a slow, gradual withdrawal. Please don't do as many women tell me they have done, which is to just get fed up and throw the prescription away all at once. Some women are fine when they do this, and it is one choice among many. Going off hormones all at once may be easy for one woman and horrible for another. It boils down to knowing oneself.

Because you are taking herbs and not hormone stimulants as you slowly decrease estrogen, the relative drop in estrogen will mean that sometimes there is no buildup of the uterine lining. For that reason, if you have a uterus and if you have been used to having a monthly release of blood, don't worry when it skips and ends. If you are concerned about this, consult with a trusted, supportive health-care provider. It is also always wise to continue regular checkups for general wellness and your own particular health concerns.

chapter 4
Postmenopause

Postmenopause is defined as the time one year after the last menstrual bleed. But it is far more than that. Margaret Mead famously said, "The most creative force in the world is the menopausal woman with zest." The cultural anthropologist was discussing her finding that the woman who is no longer having children becomes one of the "wise women" in her community. Mead also said, "Never doubt that a small group of thoughtful, committed citizens can change the world; indeed, it's the only thing that ever has." In his novel Intruders in the Dust, William Faulkner wrote that if we need an impossible task accomplished, a wrong righted, or a noble effort performed with grace and skill, we can forget about contacting elected officials, venerated city fathers, or even energetic youths. Instead, ask an older woman. There is profound truth in this observation. Older women know how to get things done. Indeed, there are many books written about the vital force of women's wisdom.

After menopause, many women find themselves moving out of an intense phase of child rearing and career building to pursue new passions and adventures. For some, it brings the freedom to accomplish deep personal transformation. Yet this vibrant third of life often comes with critical challenges, particularly in the areas of health and financial security. Many senior women fear retirement because they lack sufficient income to meet their basic needs. Loss of a life partner and distance from family members adds to the emotional and survival issues faced by older women.

Most women experience mood swings during and after menopause, and these are usually not a major health risk. Still, women are four times more likely to have symptoms, even with no previous history of depression. It never rains, but it pours: women with hot flashes are twice as likely to develop depression. Though hormones reduce this risk, it is certain now that using hormones at all increases the risk of breast cancer. Research supports the clinical experience of herbalists and naturopathic doctors, who find that women using herbal remedies for symptoms as diverse as hot flashes and depression respond well and safely over time.

Whatever your personal circumstances, your postmenopausal years offer you a new opportunity to change how you care for yourself. Herbal medicine can strengthen body, mind, and spirit to face challenges that arise, as well as to energize you to pursue new interests. Keeping active and fit supports your well-being better than anything. Natural therapies help minimize potential health problems. Buoyed by renewed energy, you can continue to meet life's challenges and thrive.

This chapter discusses herbal and other natural remedies for some of the most common health conditions affecting postmenopausal women. The herbal mixtures here, both tea blends and combined extracts, are formulated so that you can safely use the faster-acting extracts along with the milder teas without fear of overdosing. The teas are effective by themselves for long-standing conditions and may be a more affordable option.

Because more happens to us after menopause than problems with breasts and uterus, we'll begin with common and treatable joint pain.

ARTHRITIS

Arthritis is an inflammation that occurs where two bones meet in a joint. Painful joints are more than a "mechanical" annoyance: they are especially hard to cope with when the hands are affected or when pain in the knees and hips makes exercise difficult to enjoy. Arthritis is linked to insomnia, stress, other physical changes, and depression.

Depression is commonly undiagnosed when it is combined with arthritis. After menopause, the question is, do hormonal changes cause depression, or does depression alter the action of hormones? Making it still more complex for allopathic medicine to target, providers must determine whether the arthritic change associated with aging is responsible for the depression, or whether the effect of stress, anxiety, and depression is more inflammation and thus more sedentary habits.

There are two main types of arthritis: wear-and-tear arthritis, or *osteoarthritis*, and the autoimmune type, *rheumatoid arthritis*. Osteoarthritis, associated with years of repeated physical movement that wears some joints out faster than others, usually affects joints in the hips, shoulders, fingers, and neck. In osteoarthritis, there is a loss of the glassy-smooth cartilage where two bones meet, so the bones rub against each other. The body responds by making the whole area stiff, swollen, red, and sore in the hope it will be rested instead of stressed further. Although injury or sports may worsen the condition, so will inactivity: surrounding muscles contract, further drawing the bones close up against each other. Obesity is an important cause as well. When they rub, the friction causes more heat. Damp weather also causes muscle contraction and can worsen the condition, as can stress, which may be reflected in unconscious tension placed on joints and other vulnerable spots in the body. The following formulas therefore contain herbs that relax muscle tension.

Rheumatoid arthritis usually starts as an illness accompanied by fevers and joint pain that moves around the body or comes and goes. Because this form of arthritis isn't due to wear and tear but is in the bloodstream, it may hit non-weight-bearing joints and the same joints on both sides of the body (both elbows, both thumbs, and so forth). It may coexist with other autoimmune conditions.

The cause of rheumatoid arthritis (RA) is debated, but it is classed as an autoimmune disorder. The idea is that immune cells consider the cells lining the joints to be foreign invaders, so they attack them, resulting in inflammation, pain, and stiffness. This notion is being revised in light of information about molecular mimicry, when microbes mimic cells our body knows as "self." The presence of infective microbes such as campylobacter and shigella found in RA patients is altering the way the medical community views the cause and treatment of this class of diseases. Like all autoimmune conditions, rheumatoid arthritis is complex enough for a woman to seek professional health care, but the following recommendations will improve it and are unlikely to make it worse.

You can have both types of arthritis, because autoimmune destruction of a joint can lead to wear and tear. Though family history may be associated with these diseases, you don't automatically inherit them just because a parent or grandparent has joint problems. Diagnosis in both cases is confirmed by X-rays and blood tests. If you have arthritis or think you are a candidate for it, you need to be especially careful to control body fat. The five to ten extra pounds or so that women usually gain after menopause are protective, provided they are composed of a mixture of muscle and dense bone. These tissues develop from exercising. A little cushioning of fat under the skin helps maintain our internal balance of estrogen and protects us in case we take a tumble. Exercise additionally helps by improving coordination even when joints are stiff and aching. Walking speed is a simple and reliable measure of how we function in health as we age. A study that included more than thirteen thousand postmenopausal women (mostly age sixty-five) from the Women's Health Initiative started with women who had not had a stroke, though later, 264 did have a stroke. The other factors this study took into account included the women's ages, race/ethnicity, body mass index, waist-hip ratio, depression, arthritis, hypertension, smoking, systolic blood pressure, treated diabetes, hormone use, NSAID use, aspirin use, self-reported general health, and history of coronary heart disease. Not only was walking found to be protective, but researchers also found that slower walking speed was a "significant predictor" of stroke. Stretching or enjoying yoga designed for elders can safely return freedom of movement to your body. Eating foods naturally high in anti-inflammatory compounds is another way to protect your heart and your joints.

Neck stiffness caused by arthritis can lead to frequent headaches, but you should avoid the temptation to take aspirin or painkillers regularly. Frequent use can eventually damage the stomach lining, reduce liver cell function, and worsen ringing in your ears (called tinnitus). The natural salicylates found in willow and meadowsweet were originally the source of aspirin, but the herb teas are not concentrated enough for some headaches. However, the herbs are far better for joints and heart health, and may prevent future headaches. Postmenopausal women (or any midlife woman) with frequent or severe headaches is best evaluated by a professional to rule out other causes such as inflamed arteries (arteritis), a risk for cerebrovascular disease.

Although dietary changes, exercise, and herbal preparations cannot always reverse changes to bone tissue, they can reduce the severity of arthritic symptoms. The following herbal formulas can help clear the body of inflammatory "junk" that triggers flare-ups. Because pain and other body changes related to arthritis may well bring on depression, some of the herbs traditionally used for arthritic pain, swelling, and stiffness are also relaxing yet mood lifting. While media attention on the popular herb black cohosh has raged pro and con, the traditional use of the herb has been confirmed by most researchers as both effective within specific dosage ranges and safe. The confusion arises in part because many positive human trials, and some with conflicting data, are bedeviled by a lack of certainty about how black cohosh works to relieve menopausal symptoms. Once believed to be a phytoestrogen, black cohosh root was later reclassified as a SERM (selective estrogen receptor modifier). It may act this way in the brain, bone, and vaginal canal. This would explain why black cohosh is often shown to improve hot flashes, bone density, and mood. Still later, concerns about liver toxicity were raised as a possible problem, but these fears were resolved in the herb's favor by researchers in 2004. These researchers and others have published a study proposing that serotonin-like activity might explain some of the herb's potency, at least in test tubes. This makes sense, because serotonin receptors in the body are involved in temperature control and sensitivity to hot flashes. Because the effect appears to be centrally mediated, the herb does not cause problems in breast and uterine tissue as estrogen does. At the time of this writing, there are more than eighty-five papers and presentations on the safety and efficacy of standardized black cohosh.

Traditional northeastern First Nations used decoctions (teas) of black cohosh roots for aching joints, especially during cold wet seasons, for midlife people of both genders. Another herb well covered in the media, St. John's wort, is not the dangerous weed it has been painted to be in less-informed circles. Long before its use to treat depression, St. John's wort was enjoyed as a restorative to nerves after damage (wear-and-tear arthritis or trauma). The concern with herb-drug interaction has been limited in a recent analysis of older studies to two groups: those on HIV drugs, such as the antiretroviral zidovudine, and transplant patients on the immune suppressant cyclosporine. Both these treatments for these particular patients are under review for advances in these fields. The ability of St. John's wort to speed the liver's breakdown of the drugs makes sense, since it is used to help the liver's primary function of detoxification and clearance of foreign substances.

Herbal Medicine

Boswellia carterii, commonly called frankincense, is described in Exodus in the Old Testament. This resinous tree sap was used historically and still is today as a universal remedy for infection, bleeding, and pain of muscle, tendon, and joints. Frankincense came to the holy land via the famous spice route across southern Arabia and east Africa, the same caravan highway used for goods from India and the East. Some frankincense still comes from Arabia, but most frankincense today comes from Somalia (among the leading exports, it is third after bananas and cattle). Its cultivation, harvesting, and international marketing provides work for some ten thousand Somali families. Most goes to Saudi Arabia, Yemen, and Egypt, the major markets, but its use for two autoimmune conditions, ulcerative colitis and RA, have increased sales in Europe and North America. The best way to take Boswellia is in coated tablets or capsules of concentrated extract, not just powdered herb. The effective dose is between 400 and 1,200 milligrams three times a day, with concentrations of boswellic acid anywhere from 37 percent in some products to 70 percent in others. However, the acid concentration is only one marker of an effective extract of the whole herb, and the correct dose depends on other factors. The following formula aims at a lower dose to synergize with other herbs and to prevent the stomach upset that sometimes comes with use of resinous plants. The reason why Boswellia is particularly useful here in that it reduces inflammation in joints as well as speeding tissue repair in the digestive tract. Many health-care providers of integrative medicine find a strong association between success with joint pain and restoring integrity to the digestive system. How the herb works has to do with its effects on two enzymes with the long names of cyclo-oxygenase 1 and

2 (COX-1, COX-2). COX-1 helps protect and maintain several types of tissue. COX-2 governs inflammation, a normal response to stress or injury, but in arthritis and chronic inflammation, a cause of pain. Boswellia inhibits this enzyme, with effects on related compounds such as leukotrienes, thus reducing inflammation and pain. Unlike the COX-2-inhibiting drugs for pain (such as Vioxx, pulled from the market in 2004 after it was found to worsen heart health and increase risk of stroke), Boswellia is a safe anti-inflammatory with a long history of human use. Clinical trials of standardized extracts have not revealed any serious side effects, though its safety in therapeutic doses has not been set for young children or pregnant women. However, since it is a resin, there is always the possibility of a mild upset stomach, even though human trials have shown Boswellia helps with ulcerative colitis, Crohn's disease, and other inflammatory, painful conditions. Other medicinal plants known to share this COX-2-inhibiting effect are turmeric (*Curcuma longa*), ginger (*Zingiber officinale*), and hops (*Humulus lupulus*), and the compound resveratrol (found in grape seeds and other herbs).

Concentrate for joint health

CONCENTRATED HERB EXTRACT	ACTIONS
4 oz. willow bark *(Salix alba)*	Reduces inflammation, pain
3 oz. frankincense *(Boswellia carterii)*	Cox-2 inhibitor; pain-reducing anti-inflammatory
3 oz. St. John's wort herb *(Hypericum perforatum)*	Antidepressant; repairs nerves; strengthens immunity
1 oz. alfalfa leaf *(Medicago sativa)*	Nutritive; antiarthritic; provides minerals
2 oz. black cohosh root *(Cimicifuga racemosa)*	Antiarthritic; relaxes nerves; hormonal tonic

Combine these herbal extracts. Take 1 teaspoon in 1 cup of water, juice, or any herb tea in the morning and evening. Allow thirty days for best effects, though improvement may be felt in a couple of days.

Twelve ounces will last thirty days.

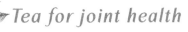
Tea for joint health

DRIED HERBS	ACTIONS
2 oz. willow bark (*Salix alba*)	Reduces inflammation; improves elimination through kidneys
3 oz. meadowsweet herb (*Filipendula ulmaria*)	Anti-inflammatory; heals stomach lining; for taste
1 oz. St. John's wort herb (*Hypericum perforatum*)	Antidepressant; repairs nerves; strengthens immunity
1 oz. alfalfa leaf (*Medicago sativa*)	Nutritive; antiarthritic; provides minerals

Add ½ ounce of the mixture to 3½ cups of boiling water in a teapot or container with a well-fitting lid. Let stand for fifteen minutes before straining. Drink 1 cup, hot or cold, three times a day. If you prefer, sip tea all day or drink two large glasses twice a day, making sure you drink 3 cups a day.

Seven ounces will last about fourteen days.

There is a more complicated recipe for an elixir, in which some herbs are extracted in water, others in alcohol, and all are mixed together for a long-lasting remedy taken in small daily doses over several months to a year. It is no more difficult than making lasagna or a cherry pie, though the steps may at first seem difficult because the ingredients may be unfamiliar. My favorite elixir for long-standing joint pain that affects several areas of the body is on page 121.

Nutrition

Review the following suggestions for whole foods that provide vitamins and minerals to address joint health.

wise food choices

❋ ORAC (oxygen radical absorbance capacity) foods are high in their ability to eradicate free radicals. These include many fruits, berries, grapes, and other plants. The research suggests mixing them rather than relying on one or two to produce the best effects for longevity.

(ORAC units per 100 grams—about 3.5 ounces)
Açai berries: more than 10,000
Prunes: 5,770 (these are also noted in research for their value in improving bone density)
Raisins: 2,830
Blueberries: 2,400 to more than 9,000
Blackberries: 2,036

Kale: 1,770
Strawberries: 1,540
Raspberries: 1,220
Brussels sprouts: 980
Plums: 949
Alfalfa sprouts: 930
Broccoli florets: 890
Beets: 840
Oranges: 750
Cherries: 670
Onion: 450
Corn: 400

❋ Include the warming spices, turmeric and ginger root, in vegetable and protein dishes to your taste preference. These are rich in antioxidants that have anti-inflammatory properties.

❋ Eat steamed dark green vegetables at least twice a week, but avoid spinach, rhubarb, and other oxalate-containing vegetables and fruits.

❋ Limit or avoid alcohol, because it is a depressant and contributes to some women's arthritis. If you want a glass of wine at dinner to help digestion or sleep, avoid red wine because red grape products worsen arthritis. For this reason, also avoid red grapes, red wine vinegar, and purple grape juice. As a general rule, alcohol should not be used as a sleep aid because it seems to help at first, only to lead to rebound wakefulness.

❋ Consider food allergies for a trial of elimination and challenge. In naturopathy and many systems of medical herbal therapy, joint pain is viewed as having its roots in digestive disturbances. Food allergies are not always to blame, while misconceptions about genuine food allergies abound in mainstream culture. A simple way to develop a sense for whether your immune system reacts to common foods with symptoms of joint pain is to avoid them. The following are among the most frequently identified food triggers to exclude:

Sugar and all processed food
Grains, starting with wheat
Dairy, alcohol, caffeine, red meat
Potato, tomato, eggplant

Avoid these long enough to give the immune system a rest from hyperarousal (three weeks each). That is only practical for most people when they rotate through an elimination diet. First, exclude sugars, which most of us do not need even after a three-week break. Next, cut out grains for three weeks, especially if you live on whole wheat sandwiches. Cycle through the other foods, giving each one a good span of time before you reintroduce it. After three weeks off red meat, eating a steak either causes a return of symptoms within one or two days, or it doesn't.

❋ Even without food allergies, you can reduce pain in joints by limiting or avoiding coffee (decaffeinated or regular), dairy products (from cows, especially milk, cheese, and butter), potatoes, tomatoes, eggplants, cayenne pepper, black pepper, and bell or green peppers.

- ✿ Eat unprocessed, high-quality foods, organic if possible.

- ✿ As an anti-inflammatory and diuretic, try celery as an unlimited raw vegetable (organic tastes good, commercial tastes boring), and its seeds in cooking, or freshly juiced. In herbal medicine, the term explaining celery's action for people with arthritis is alterative. This means it is a gentle nutritive that alters a long-standing condition such as arthritis.

- ✿ Eat something raw every day (a salad in summer, an apple in colder weather).

- ✿ Eat complex carbohydrates in moderation (gluten-free buckwheat, quinoa, possibly rice).

- ✿ Prefer vegetarian protein or cold-water fish over pork, beef, and dairy.

- ✿ Drink one quart or more of herb tea or filtered water every day.

supplements

- ✿ Optimize your omega-3 and omega-6 essential fatty acid intake. GLA is short for gamma-linoleic acid found in evening primrose oil, while EPA is eicopentasoic acid found in cold-water fish such as salmon and herring. Flaxseed provides omega-3 oil and is standard medical therapy from European doctors after any heart attack. Aim for 1 to 3 grams daily.

- ✿ Try SAM-e, S-adenosylmethionine; the dose of this supplement to optimize both mood and joints depends on the quality. Since it degrades (becomes less potent) easily, SAM-e is best in blister packs (where you push tablets from a foil-lined pouch or "blister"), in 400-milligram doses.

- ✿ Try glucosamine (from shellfish; 2000 milligrams per day) and chondroitin (from cartilage; 1200 milligrams per day).

In Addition

- ✿ The essential oil of bay makes a fine massage blend, though undiluted it may be too strong. Add five or six drops to an ounce of safflower or any vegetable oil, and rub it into painful joints, especially the small joints of the hands and feet.

- ✿ Add ten drops of lavender essential oil to a comfortably hot bath; swish the water to disperse the oil. Light a candle in a safe place, close the door, and soak your bones, smoothing the lavender water into your skin. Skip the soap tonight; relax for at least twenty minutes. If you've had an active day, let out the water and start a new bath as many times as you wish, until your toes and fingers "prune." Finish with a lukewarm or cool shower, and move slowly: the heat dilates blood vessels, causing some sensitive women to feel dizzy if they stand or exit the tub too quickly. If you have high blood pressure, avoid extremes of temperature and use common sense.

- ✿ To relieve pain in hands and wrists, find a salad bowl or a large, shallow container that you can easily fit your hands into. In this bowl, stir a tablespoon of dried yellow mustard powder and a little warm water into a paste. Keep adding comfortably hot water, about 4 cups (1 quart),

Elixir for healthy joints

Glass container(s) to store 5 or 6 quarts of finished elixir; for example, two sterilized apple juice gallon-size jars with well-fitting lids
5 cups (2½ pounds)of either honey or vegetable glycerin
750 ml 190-proof alcohol (unflavored) (approximately 27 to 28 fl. oz.)

DRIED HERBS	ACTIONS
Group 1	
1 oz. holy wood, lignum vitae resin, or stem bark (*Guaiacum officinale, G. sanctum*)	Antimicrobial, anti-inflammatory
2 oz. devil's claw root (*Harpagophytum procumbens*)	Anti-inflammatory
2 oz. prickly ash bark (*Zanthoxylum americanum*)	Nonheating circulation support, immune function
2 oz. willow bark (*Salix alba*)	Anti-inflammatory
4 oz. bogbean (*Menyanthes trifoliatum*)	Anti-inflammatory
4 oz. Oregon grape bark (*Mahonia aquifolium*)	Antimicrobial, clears lungs
Group 2	
2 oz. celery seed (*Apium graveolens*)	Clears uric acid via kidneys
2 oz. yarrow flowers, leaves (*Achillea millefolium*)	Anti-inflammatory, gastrointestinal support for other herbs
3 oz. angelica root (*Angelica archangelica*)	Antimicrobial, modulates immune function

In 6 quarts of water, bring the first group of herbs (15 ounces) to a boil. Immediately decrease the heat to low and simmer, covered, for 2 hours.

After 2 hours, turn off the heat, and add the second group of three herbs (7 ounces).

Let cool for 30 minutes, then stir in the honey. Cover and let steep for 4 hours or up to overnight (10 hours). Do not let the mixture stand longer than 15 hours before straining, or cover with an airtight lid and refrigerate until ready to strain.

Strain through unbleached muslin or cheesecloth into a sterilized container.

Add 16 percent alcohol by volume to discourage mold. Based on the usual yield of 5½ quarts or 175 ounces, 16 percent of 190-proof alcohol is 28 ounces.

The elixir is about 12 percent alcohol, similar to wine.

The dose is 1 tablespoon in the morning and 1 tablespoon in the afternoon for 10 weeks, then 1 tablespoon every other day or once a week for maintenance, or more frequently as needed during flare-ups or changes in weather.

squishing out lumps as you turn the paste into a thin, watery broth. Place your hands in the bowl of hot mustard water and soak them for ten to twenty minutes, occasionally adding a little more mustard powder broth or hot water to keep the hand bath comfortably hot when it cools down. After the first five minutes, begin to open and close your fists, massaging painful knuckles and joints, until swelling and stiffness have lessened and movement is easier. Rinse with lukewarm, plain water and pat (do not rub) dry. Your hands should tingle. You can repeat the treatment daily for a week or until internal remedies begin to make it less necessary. Do not use with open cuts, burns, or skin rashes; mustard can be irritating.

❀ You can purchase or make a cayenne ointment and massage it into larger areas, such as the hips, knees, and lower back. Alternatively, massage the area for ten minutes or more with 1 ounce almond oil and ¼ ounce essential oil of wintergreen. Methyl salicylate, commonly available at drugstores, is not as nice smelling but may be effective also.

❀ What about DMSO (dimethyl sulfoxide)? This antioxidant, anti-inflammatory chemical may be pain relieving, but its use is controversial. For some, it is a lifesaver; for others, it may stop being effective or may have side effects. It smells like garlic, which you may consider a disadvantage. A 70-percent DMSO, 30-percent water solution has been shown, at least in laboratory studies, to cut pain by blocking a certain type of peripheral nerve that senses pain, called C fibers. Clinical trials have demonstrated its effectiveness, but these were done some time ago. More recent research has focused on the role of DMSO in treating cancer cells or its uses in industry. It has its fans, but because DMSO is not an herb, I have not used this compound in my practice.

❀ Therapeutic sweats are a traditional way to rejuvenate a tired body. Contact health spas or saunas in your local area; ask personnel for information about the cautions and benefits of steam rooms or hot tubs.

❀ Any amount of exercise helps, no matter how little you think you can do. Especially healing are activities involving slow movement: tai chi, stretching, swimming, yoga, and dance. Be sure to let the class instructor know your interest, level of fitness, and special concerns. Remember that unaccustomed new movements may work muscles you have forgotten about and cause soreness, but if you do not feel better soon, find a more receptive teacher.

❀ Mind-body approaches can make this part of your life easier. Filtering thoughts that value only youth can prevent self-judgment about feeling exactly as you do now. Actively stop yourself from saying, *This is awful.* Ask yourself, *What do I want? What is in store in this next phase of my life?* Build in time with women and friends of any age. Sharing laughs makes your experience less awful and more amenable to self-help.

❀ Try the Joint Mobility Visualization (see page 123).

CHANGING NUTRITIONAL NEEDS

You keep up with health news—but what if you can't stand soy, or it makes you feel bloated? You may find that you can't eat salads anymore without suffering from indigestion. Indigestion from

Joint Mobility Visualization

Try the following visualization. Sit or stand, feet flat on the floor, weight distributed evenly. Imagine yourself just as you are. Pressing your shoulders back and dropping them down, breathe in and out evenly and slowly. See your bones as levers. Imagine that when they move they are pulling muscles. For five or ten minutes, picture your muscles smoothly and comfortably performing the movements you make each day. Visualize your movements as realistically as you can. Perhaps you see yourself picking something up from the floor, reaching up to close a window. If you wince when you imagine any movement, take a slow breath, count to ten, and then imagine it again in slow motion, visualizing it as effortless movement, even if it is a different reach or stretch. Straighten your spine to lengthen it a few inches while you continue to breathe. Stretch your hands out and make fists, then relax them. Allow your vision to clear so you can know the image of the body you already have within yourself waiting to be realized. If you are sitting, rise as slowly as you can, concentrating only on feeling the subtle changes you have already begun to visualize in your mind.

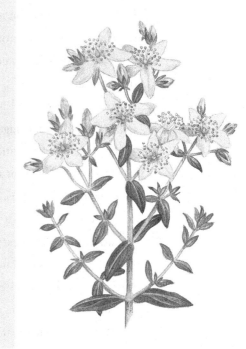

lettuce and other "health" foods may be traced to low levels of stomach acid, which must be produced in sufficient quantity to break down roughage. The difficulty with digestion during and after menopause is the accursed gassiness. We also need stomach acid to extract vitamins and minerals from the indigestible cellulose of plant foods. But why do many older women have low stomach acid? Some functions decline with age, but we are designed to keep eating and digesting food without buying enzymes, as useful as they sometimes are. Loading up on calcium carbonate and chalky dolomite supplements for ten or fifteen years is one possible explanation for low stomach acid; consumption of calcium-rich antacid tablets is another.

Nevertheless, not all women who experience indigestion take calcium supplements, so every case can't be the fault of supplements alone. Although efficient digestion gradually decreases with aging, many of the modern Western digestive problems we suffer from have as much to do with the chemically treated, factory-farm produce generally available. Farmers' markets and other local food (ideally, growing your own!) are the way to go. Lightly steam fresh vegetables to make them more digestible, and switch among various kinds of staples such as whole grains to reduce dependence on wheat.

One way to improve nutrition as you age is to rekindle a strong digestive metabolism with nutritive herbs and vegetables. These plants, called "bitters," also help stabilize blood sugar by stimulating the mobilization of proteins and sugars stored in the pancreas, liver, and blood. Certain bitter herbs such as dandelion root and leaf can help women control adult-onset (Type 2) diabetes. Other herbs with a mild to strong bitter flavor (radicchio in salads or the potent *Andrographis paniculata* as tablets) can help women with low blood sugar control their cravings for refined sugar. Because diabetes can worsen with age or multiple medications, every healthy technique you can use to avoid increased need for oral hypoglycemics is worth practicing. For insulin-dependent diabetes, close monitoring of blood sugar changes and checking with your physician are always recommended.

Your changing nutritional needs and digestive capacity may cause unexpected symptoms such as constipation. This is not a failure of your body; rather, it may be your body's healthy signal that you must eat differently now. The three most natural remedies for irregular bowel elimination are movement (walking), fiber (fruit, vegetables, grains), and increased water. For some women, though, it is hard to force down extra water or liquids. Since the 1930s the common advice has been to drink six to eight glasses of water a day. Yet some women are going to feel inadequate, even guilty, if they can't manage this because of urinary frequency. Eating more soups and fewer animal proteins is one way to ease the burden.

The digestive tea that follows contains herbs that will get the old digestive motors up and running. It's an all-around blend for many minor digestive symptoms; drinking ½ cup before or after meals will stimulate the liver to regulate nutrient balance and bowel function. A final note on constipation: avoid regular use of herbal laxatives that irritate the colon (senna and *Cascara sagrada*). These are particularly bad if you are trying to lose weight, because emptying the colon is not the same as burning off unwanted fat. The occasional use of laxatives to relieve constipation for one or two nights at a time can be helpful, but don't use them unless they're really needed.

When food is not digested well, this creates "bad" bacteria in your stomach; the bacteria throw a party and then leave you to deal with the consequences—more gas. Whether particular foods, genetic predisposition, or something as yet unclear to us is responsible, the answer is to eat differently. As with blood sugar and constipation, bitter salad vegetables (such as endive and chicory) stimulate peristalsis, combined with gas-reducing aromatic herbs such as fennel seeds, thyme, and rosemary. Small pinches of the slightly bitter Mexican herb epazote (*Chenopodium ambrosioides*) cooked with each standard size pot of beans helps reduce flatulence. Avoid foods that cause gas and bloating such as cabbage and cheese. Include in recipes any of the pleasant-tasting, volatile oil–containing herbs—for example, cinnamon, sage, and other favorite culinary herbs—to clear out the bulk of the bad bacteria. These tend to be herbs that add spice to dishes and sweeten the breath. The best is parsley (always organic, to avoid pesticide residues in those leafy folds). You can take the following concentrate or tea after heavy meals to settle digestive upsets, clear intestinal gas, and nourish the body parts that nourish you.

Herbal Medicine

Concentrate for digestive strength

CONCENTRATED HERB EXTRACT	ACTIONS
2 oz. peppermint leaf (*Mentha piperita*)	Antiseptic; kills bad bacteria, reduces gas
2 oz. lemon balm leaf (*Melissa officinalis*)	Lifts spirits, reduces bloating; antiviral
1 oz. chamomile flower (*Matricaria recutita*)	Soothes nerves, quiets intestinal spasms

Combine these extracts. Take 1 to 2 teaspoons diluted in 1 cup of water after or between meals, as needed, up to three times a day. If you are allergic to chrysanthemum flowers or chamomile itself, leave them out.

Five ounces will last ten days of regular use, or longer if used occasionally.

Tea for digestive strength

DRIED HERBS	ACTIONS
2 oz. peppermint leaf (*Mentha piperita*)	Antiseptic; kills bad bacteria, reduces gas
2 oz. lemon balm leaf (*Melissa officinalis*)	Lifts spirits, reduces bloating; antiviral
1 oz. chamomile flower (*Matricaria recutita*)	Soothes nerves, quiets intestinal spasms

For quick relief, add 1 ounce of the combination to 2 to 3 cups of boiling water in a teapot with a well-fitting lid or other covered container. Let sit for fifteen minutes; strain and drink ½ cup before each meal and ½ cup afterward up to four times a day for five days. For occasional need or for use as an enjoyable digestive beverage, add 1 to 2 teaspoons of this mixture to 1 cup of boiling water and leave covered for ten to fifteen minutes, then strain and drink as desired. Best after or between meals, as needed, up to three times each day.

Five ounces will last five to ten days of regular use, or longer if used occasionally.

A note about weight gain: it is usual, no matter how little you eat, to experience some weight gain postmenopausally. However, be aware that a waist size greater than thirty-five inches around at the navel is strongly linked to insulin resistance. The answer to keeping blood sugar and other measures of health (such as resistance to infections) in balance is simple. Reduce your amount of calories per day by 200. Exercise more, even if it is walking just a little farther than the day before. Over time, gravity pulls us into a potentially charming pear shape even if we keep active. For some of us, the thighs thicken no matter how much we exercise. For many women, the problem with this change isn't the weight per se. It is the rapid weight gain in fat, as opposed to muscle weight, that makes us feel bad—both because of how our bodies feel and because we are somehow not conforming to our culture's standard, preferred image of health and attractiveness. Well, I say to hell with that. It's time the sick culture that undervalues wisdom in our elders starts conforming to our healthy standards of self-image. Women writing on the subject of health today describe a range of new norms that are as numerous as the stars you can see in a rural night sky. Women who reject the stereotypes of attracting either sex as the point of life might find it satisfying to focus on the inner work of the spirit or work out in the world. Let any changes in weight that you experience direct you to your perfect path, whether weight management be through working out in a gym or a garden, joining an agit-prop theater group, or finding your strength on a yoga mat.

Overweight is defined as a basal metabolic index (BMI) of obesity is 30kg/m^2. One kilogram is 2.2 pounds—divide your weight in pounds by 2.2 to know your weight in kilos. Your BMI equals weight in kilograms divided by height in meters squared. Too much math? There are some easy-to-use BMI calculators on the Internet. You know if you need to trim down or shape up, anyway. Ideal weights are usually defined by height, weight, and daily calorie expenditure. The range for each of us is relatively easy to discover, either by asking a health-care provider or figuring it out ourselves from books, websites, and common sense. The epidemic of obesity in the mainstream culture is not due to ignorance of ideal weights for individuals, but because many people just won't exercise and eat better.

One way to deal with weight gain is to exercise daily or weekly over the months and years, so that the weight is added in the form of dense bone, muscle, and only a little extra fat. Also, be your own advocate for your health and self-image. To do so, you will need to reevaluate your own needs and reality and dismiss other people's prejudices. Do you need to lose some weight to lessen the strain on your heart or arthritic bones? Or is this the time to loosen up about your waistline and accept yourself as you are? Only you can decide. Beware of easy, feel-good answers that are not your truth. While women who are more trim have less risk of heart disease and diabetes, for instance, the goal is health, not being skinny at all costs. The other extreme of ignoring weight gain isn't doing women any good. It is not "feminist" to be unhealthy and risk a heart attack just because the dominant society sells products using male-oriented sexual imagery. Remaining overweight as a protest against society or as protection against sexual advances does not gain us equal rights. Only self-knowledge and free choice can do that, whatever the scales say.

Be wary, too, of herb products or diets promising quick results. Only through slow, careful self-care—plus exercising your choice of foods that nourish the emerging potential—can you build vital energy, endurance, and reliable results that last. If I could outlaw harmful foods that heartless corporations get rich on, I would. But that would not stop obesity any more than outlawing drugs has stopped humans' urge to get high. Obesity is not the fault of the dreadful food that exists in mainstream culture; rather, it's the fault of our willingness to think that processed garbage is food.

"If you take in more calories than you burn you gain weight." The conventional view is that biology works on a simple basis—what goes in and doesn't get used turns to fat. But this doesn't take into account all the factors, including the role of the marketing of harmful nonfoods and then the marketing of pills to take off weight.

Drugs intended for short-term use—under three months—are supposed to be available only from doctors, but are available cheaply online. These are phentermine (which causes side effects, mainly insomnia, in one out of ten people) and similar drugs that increase levels of the neurotransmitter serotonin. Increased serotonin may decrease cravings for fat or carbohydrates, but studies show we cannot rely on this. Also, these drugs may not increase basal metabolic rate (BMR) but may help food be metabolized better.

Antidepressant drugs that work this way—selective serotonin reuptake inhibitors (SSRIs)—are also used, but studies show they help weight loss at six months yet cannot guarantee lasting change at one year, and they may even cause weight gain. Also, cholesterol-lowering drugs are sometimes prescribed to decrease fat absorption, but these may interfere with nutrient absorption.

Research shows that the glycemic index (GI) of foods is not the key to lasting weight loss. Conducted at the Jean Mayer U.S. Department of Agriculture Human Nutrition Research Center on Aging (USDA HNRCA) at Tufts University, a 2008 study looked at the relationship between calorie-restricted diets, aging, and age-related disease. The first phase of the study, which was conducted over a period of twelve months, revealed that calorie-restricted diets differing substantially in glycemic load can result in comparable long-term weight loss. "Participants in our pilot study achieved and maintained comparable weight loss after one year, regardless of whether they were on a low-glycemic-load or a high-glycemic-load diet," said Dr. Susan Roberts, director of the USDA HNRCA's Energy Metabolism Laboratory. "The goal was for both groups to restrict calories by 30 percent and, after one year, both groups had lost an average of 8 percent of their original body weight. We found that the two groups did not differ significantly in their average body fat loss, energy intake, metabolic rate, or reports of hunger and satiety."

Although the glycemic index (GI) has been around for twenty years, initially intended as a guideline for diabetics, it has been used to give a marketing edge to many foods since 2003. It is of value, but more important perhaps is the rate at which natural plant sugars from carrots and corn are released into the bloodstream as the digestive tract liberates these carbohydrates from the fiber in all vegetables, fruits, and grains.

The following herbal recommendations are not a quick-weight-loss formula. Their purpose is to stabilize a woman's total health. You may find that they reduce food cravings and gas; in addition, they increase nutrition during changes in eating and exercising. The first recipe here is high in caffeine, antioxidants, and non-caffeine herbs that support healthy nerves and immunity.

Herbal Medicine

Tea for increasing metabolism

CONCENTRATED HERB EXTRACT	ACTIONS
4 oz. yerba mate (*Ilex paraguaensis*)	Caffeine; reduces physical and mental fatigue; improves nonspecific immunity
½ oz. guarana (*Paullinia cupana*)	Caffeine; nervine stimulant
4 oz. damiana (*Turnera diffusa*)	Mild antidepressant; digestive aid; mild diuretic; flavor
1½ oz. green tea (*Camellia sinensis*)	Antioxidant; immune protective; lowers blood lipids; prevents tooth decay; increases basic metabolic rate (BMR); flavor

Steep 1 tablespoon in 1½ cups of boiling water for twenty minutes; strain out the tea leaves. Sip 1 cup up to 4 cups per day for three weeks as part of a kick-start to weight management.

Use less or discontinue use if you are sensitive to caffeine or develop headaches, a racing heart, or poor sleep. Sleep disturbances can, and often do, happen during and after menopause, even if caffeine is taken as long as ten to twelve hours before bedtime. A caffeine-free herbal recipe follows on page 130.

How long the tea blend lasts depends on how many cups a day you feel you need. If it tastes at all bitter or sour, use far less. This blend works when it tastes pleasant and is taken consistently over time, with no side effects such as jittery nerves.

Though it contains caffeine, yerba mate prevents stress on the heart, and preliminary reports suggest that it may repair damaged DNA. The herb contains vitamins A, E, B complex, and C. In addition, it contains fifteen different amino acids and significant amounts of magnesium, calcium, iron, sodium, potassium, manganese, phosphates, zinc, niacin, sulfur, chlorophyll, choline, and inositol. Tiny amounts of some constituents are in the herb; some of those same minerals and plant chemicals are used as supplements for weight loss.

An obese person who drops fifteen pounds also drops her risk of disease because if the fat was centered around the waistline, the body loses fat from organs such as the liver first. Yet in other situations, the scale can't tell you whether lost body weight was fat, lean muscle mass, or water (as is common with high-protein diets). Though scales are a useful guide, they have their limits. Losing weight is dull. On the other hand, gaining fitness feels like something to enjoy for the rest of your life.

Looking at the science of weight loss, we can see that natural appetite suppressants—those that do not kill us off as a way of losing weight—target the hypothalmus, creating healthy communication among various organs, systems, and neurotransmitters such as serotonin.

Ginger may help weight loss. Long used to improve digestion and circulation, regular use of ginger stimulates the pancreas and other digestive structures to make more enzymes. Ginger tea reduces blood fats even after eating a meal rich in fats. Long-term use of ginger in food and tea has been shown to be safe. We have familiarity with ginger from centuries of human use in India, China, and Southeast Asia. Besides its well-known effect on reducing nausea, ginger slows gastric emptying, so the same meal makes you feel full longer and your gut has more time to extract the nutrients without spiking blood sugar.

Hoodia is a fat-fighting herb of celebrity status. Physically lean bushmen of African regions where the succulent plant grows use it when food is scarce, but it is now endangered, on the CITES list. Namibian growers have joined together to protect the quality of exports and growers. Independent herbal researchers have found it is so limited as a raw supply that substitutions in the market are common. Instead of grabbing for the weight loss herb of the moment, remember that you deserve to love yourself and find your beauty and happiness within. This is not a competition; it is the time on the planet that you were given to live. Whether it's five pounds you want to lose or two hundred, your past does not have to be your potential.

A formula without caffeine that may serve you works on resetting the self-governance of metabolism while initiating a gentle cleanse. It is easiest to combine these as prepared tinctures in the following proportions, but a capsule or tea blend is also effective. Three #00 size capsules before meals three times a day is an approximate equivalent. As tea, there is no study to back up this dose, but an educated guess would be to steep 1 ounce of the blend in 3 to 4 cups of water just off the boil, covered for twenty minutes; drink a full cup before meals three times a day. A minimum length of time to observe metabolic change from any preparation of the following formula is likely to be upward of six weeks. If you are on any other medications, the desired metabolic shift is something for which you and your care provider can be prepared. Banaba leaf, for instance, is available in many forms, usually a 30- to 45-milligram dose standardized to 1 percent corsolic acid, and human trials demonstrate safety except in pregnancy or for children. Yet at the time of this writing, no dose has been proven to be *the* effective dose.

A caffeine-free approach for increasing metabolism

CONCENTRATED HERB EXTRACT	ACTIONS
2 oz. dandelion leaf (*Taraxacum officinale*)	Aids liver and kidneys in detoxification
2 oz. dandelion root (*Taraxacum officinale*)	Aids liver and kidneys in detoxification
2 oz. nettle leaf (*Urtica dioica*)	Aids elimination; provides energy without caffeine jitters
4 oz. banaba leaf (*Lagerstroemia speciosa*)	Stabilizes or lowers high blood sugar
⅛ oz. (or to taste) stevia (*Stevia rebaudiana*)	Herbal sweetener without calories

OPTIONAL WARMING AIDS TO DIGESTION, CIRCULATION:

¼ tsp. powdered or crushed cardamom seeds (*Elettaria cardomomum*)

½ tsp. powdered cinnamon (*Cinnamonum ceylonicum, C.* species)

½ tsp. powdered, or 1 tsp. chopped fresh ginger root (*Zingiber officinale*)

Combine these extracts and store in a dark brown or blue glass bottle with a well-fitting lid and a label. Shake well before each dose. Take 5 ml (1 teaspoon) in water before meals three times a day, for two weeks before reassessing whether to continue or not.

---

nutrition for healthy weight

❖ Apples. A clinical trial found that overweight women lost more by snacking on unlimited apples a day than on "weight loss" foods or oatmeal cookies. Organic apples are worth the extra pennies—commercial apples hold on to more pesticide residue and the peel has the magnesium, vitamin C, trace iron, and half of the apple's fiber, so you want that peel.

❖ Do you ruin exercise by overeating afterward? Carbo-loading before exercise with apples or ½ to 1 cup of unsprayed grapes or other favorite fruit in season (instead of prepared products for athletes in training) can keep you from eating 75 percent of the calories burned up.

❖ Oatmeal has some protein and plenty of the right kind of fiber to help people feel fuller longer. Add a tablespoon of dried cherries, berries, or raisins to hot cooked cereal, let dried fruit plump up before eating, and add a drizzle of fruit juice if needed. Skip the added milk and brown sugar. Eating any cooked cereal for breakfast results in a lower BMI over time. Hate oatmeal? Try bulgur or quinoa with almonds.

❖ On some mornings, start with an egg or two instead of toast, cold cereal, or cooked grains such as oatmeal or corn ("grits" in the South, "polenta" on the coasts). Studies suggest we eat up to 400 fewer calories on those days than if we started with a bagel. That adds up to about fifteen pounds a year. Don't pay extra for egg whites only unless you have a genuine and compelling reason. Good-quality whole eggs have vitamin E, which benefits every low-fat weight-loss plan, plus omega-3 essential fatty acids. Whole eggs also contain appreciable amounts of choline, which helps us use the cholesterol in whole eggs for increased energy—that means better fat metabolism. The quality issue is not only of importance to the individual's health. There is a greater community that benefits from purchasing organic, hormone-free, cage-free eggs. The sooner we put an end to factory farming, the healthier we'll all be.

❖ In cooler weather, start the day with a cup of soup or broth. Stock up on these for snacks and main meals, too, avoiding the cans loaded with salt and fat (to hide the lack of real flavor). One study showed that having two 10-ounce servings of broth or soup a day almost doubled the amount of weight lost in six months. You may choose to add the brown seaweed called *wakame* for extra metabolic power, and your own vegetables to plain broth so it fills you longer, burns fat, and feeds your energy reserves.

❖ Yogurt. The irritating ads about fitting into the bikini do not also inform us that commercial brands are loaded with corn syrup sweeteners. The frantic ad campaign to make us trust high-fructose corn syrup is a lie. Nor is that sludge of fruit at the bottom going to rescue us from a size 18 swimsuit. But calcium in plain low-fat yogurt three times a day for months increases fat burning, especially around the middle. Add fresh berries in season for a healthier immune system and clear skin. Turn a serving of plain yogurt into salad dressing or a dip for cut vegetables like jicama, with a dash of sea salt, oregano, parsley, turmeric, ginger, cayenne, and coarsely ground black pepper. Warming spices also turn on better fat metabolism. *Note:* If food sensitivity to dairy is a problem, skip this suggestion.

❖ Cauliflower and other vegetables. Eat nonstarchy, cancer-fighting cauliflower as much as you like. The folate and vitamin C also help. Steam it and mash with a clove of garlic, then add a drizzle of olive oil and a sprinkle of Parmesan. Broccoli

continued on page 132

and bok choy work, too. Rediscover raw radishes, sliced and soaked in ice water for five minutes to cut the harsher bite they sometimes have. They can be more addictive than potato chips.

❖ Salad. Iceberg lettuce is water disguised as a vegetable. But, it is crunchy and many people like it. Enjoy it if you like for its refreshing quality, as long as you don't drown it in fatty dressing, or think you're getting nutrition it doesn't actually provide when eaten by itself. Instead, emphasize romaine or other local organic salad greens and dark leafy vegetables. Eating a big plate or bowl of mixed dark greens, vegetables, and protein is a great way to eat real food until you are full. This keeps us from digging into the basket of white flour rolls when dining out or filling up on the pasta dish.

❖ Vegetarian protein. Use beans and lentils, in soups and stews, or cooked and added to salads. I add a pinch of cinnamon, epazote (from the Mexican spice aisle in your grocery store), and red pepper to reduce the gassy effects of eating beans. And a tablespoon of organic peanut butter with fresh alfalfa sprouts on whole grain bread is a great quick meal for when you're on the run—with the needed enzymes for intense protein digestion.

❖ Steamed white cod or halibut with lime or lemon is the number one most filling food. Of course, the Swedes studied this. They found that eating fish for lunch means eating 11 percent less at dinner. That's enough for some people to drop fifteen pounds in eight months. Oily fish from the coldest water also satisfies us with its intense flavor. If you can't eat fish or are worried about overfished oceans or mercury pollution, there are always alternatives that allow for vegetarian or vegan ways of eating.

❖ Nuts. Ten to twenty almonds, roasted unsalted peanuts, or raw cashews with a 10-ounce glass of water fills you up, providing protein, carbs, and fat, with fewer calories than you might guess, unless you eat great handfuls. Grind a tablespoon of flaxseeds and add to smoothies, salad dressings, or breakfast cereal. Seeds and nuts provide the most concentrated array of health-boosting nutrients, while preventing blood-sugar dips that push hungry dieters into the nearest donut shop.

The Women's Health Institute Dietary Modification Trial was designed to look at the effects over fifteen years of a low-fat diet, high in vegetables, fruits, and grains, on breast and colorectal cancers and cardiovascular disease in postmenopausal women. Women in one group were encouraged to drop their fat intake to 20 percent of total calories, replacing these calories from fat with calories from vegetables, fruits, and whole grains. The other group simply received diet-related education materials. Women in the low-fat, high-carbohydrate group lost about five pounds at the start of their diet change. The study found that this pattern did not significantly reduce rates of heart disease or colorectal cancer and only slightly reduced breast cancer incidence, but did seem to lower risk for ovarian cancer. These are complex diseases not only due to dietary fat, however. WHI project officer Jacques Rossouw, MD, of NHLBI (part of the National Institutes of Health), concludes that though the study was not a weight-loss study, a low-fat, high-carbohydrate dietary pattern may help contain the age-related rise in body weight seen in postmenopausal women.

NERVOUS SYSTEM CHANGES

Lowered estrogen after menopause can make menstrual migraines disappear, but new changes in the nervous system can dim the glorious horizon. It's a little hard to hear about the joy of later years when you haven't slept well because of worry or pain or when you're experiencing some unsettling loss of memory.

Stress seems to increase just when we would welcome a break from the pressure of meeting daily demands. Every woman past middle age has her own set of worries. We worry about our families or our lack of economic security; we care for disabled spouses and parents; we take in our grandchildren when their parents cannot care for them. Because we must take care of ourselves and others, drawing on all our inner resources, any one of these concerns may bring our own fear of illness out into the open. Loss of independence wins all the polls as the most frightening change older women face. For many of us, the loss of an extended family living nearby has added to our sense of isolation. The problem is that these bad feelings can be like a snowball rolling down a hill: they get bigger and bigger, becoming risk factors for depression and lowered immunity.

The changes in our nervous systems do not mean we are losing ourselves. Memory loss, sleep deprivation, and headaches can make anyone feel uncertain of her next move. But this can change. Whatever you have been doing in the past, get into the habits now that you wish to retain into your old age. Actively work at improving positive behaviors with counseling, meditation, or other healing ways.

One important way to cope with stress is to make a list of your problems, put them into order of priority, then list some of the things that can change them and the steps you can take without much effort. They don't have to be big steps, just little ones. Get up tomorrow and do something new or different. Prepare a nourishing meal. Call someone and go on a walk. Volunteer for something you care about. If you are a caregiver, perhaps you can get some occasional help so you can spend some quality time with yourself.

Another thing you can do is identify those things that turn over and over in your mind. You may or may not be able to resolve the dilemma, but perhaps you may eventually be able to identify it when it occurs and say to yourself, "There it is again!" Perhaps you may come to accept it or even laugh at it.

Everyone has known someone who aged well and enjoyed what life could offer. Thinking about what you admire and value about that person may suggest a new path for you to travel, a new adventure to embark on. Perhaps you have always wanted to do something but never had the time to try it. Now is the time. Women expressing fulfillment during this third of their lives all develop one underlying trait: they are models of an adventurous spirit. Curiosity does not kill the cat, contrary to the old adage. Following where your interests lead is the surest path to satisfying your need for physical and mental activity, interacting with interesting ideas or people, and enjoying self-sufficiency.

If nothing seems to work, if you feel as if you are always sad, if you don't want to leave the house, or if you are experiencing memory loss, you need to take care of yourself and get the help you need. Talk to someone: a friend, a family member, a community organization, or a trusted health-care practitioner.

Herbal Medicine

Nothing can replace your will to be well, but you can also safely and effectively use natural methods for support in coping with disrupted sleep patterns, loneliness, and a different response to stress. All the formulas in this section contain at least one herbal remedy to support the adrenal glands so they can help you cope with or adapt to stress. Despite the headlines from a few trials showing that ginkgo does not work, many more human studies have found ginkgo is safe and effective for improving mood. Herbalists use it for nerve health as well as improved circulation to the fingers, toes, and brain. Contrary to fears that its blood-thinning effects are harmful with similar medications, newer safety studies confirm that normal therapeutic doses are unlikely to cause problems. As a caution, I still recommend ginkgo be discontinued ten days before major surgery; speak with your health professional about this.

Concentrate for mental and emotional well-being

CONCENTRATED HERB EXTRACT	ACTIONS
2 oz. ginkgo leaf (*Ginkgo biloba*)	Improves memory, mood, blood vessels
1 oz. eleuthero root (*Eleuberococcus senticosus*)	Strengthens stress response, immune resistance
1 oz. skullcap herb (*Scutellaria laterifolia*)	Relaxes tension; mildly calming

Any adaptogen may be substituted for eleuthero (see note).

Combine these herbal extracts and store in a 4-ounce dark glass bottle. Take ¼ teaspoon in 1 cup of water, juice, or any herb tea three times a day with meals (before or after). This is a mild dose. If you do not notice a change after a week, increase to ½ teaspoon in 1 cup of water three times a day with meals. If needed, increase each dose to 1 teaspoon; if you are in good health, you can take a maximum of 2 teaspoons, which is equal to 1 ounce of the formula per day (divided over the day into three doses). If you prefer, put the 2 teaspoons in a full cup of hot water or tea, allow to cool for five or ten minutes, and then drink. This method allows much of the alcohol contained in the extracts to evaporate without destroying the beneficial properties of the herbs. The less alcohol the better, though it is safe to say that after this hot water precaution, the effects of the remaining alcohol are far outweighed by the benefits of the herbs. Check with your care provider if you have questions.

Four ounces will last approximately one week. This can be taken for six months; then you should reduce the dose to ¼ teaspoon or drop the remedy altogether. Many people find that the remedy's benefits last for some time after they stop taking it.

Note: When this book was first written, eleuthero was commonly called Siberian ginseng, a name still found in the literature and the marketplace. However, as a member of the ginseng family, but not the Panax genus, it is more proper to call it by its newer common name, eleuthero ("el-LOO-ther-oh"). In fact, it is now illegal to sell eleuthero mislabeled as Siberian ginseng. Other popular adaptogens for postmenopausal zest include the Ayurvedic tonic from India, shatavari (Asparagus racemosa), and another Siberian or arctic herb, one of many around the world with the common name of golden root (Rhodiola rosea). I prefer shatavari when vaginal wall thinning and dryness is bothersome; rhodiola is better for stress-related immune problems. The best results come from consistent use for a minimum of two to three months; good results occur from even short-term use (two to four weeks). A lower dose taken longer is more effective than a high dose taken short term.

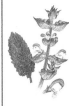

Tea for mental and emotional well-being

DRIED HERBS	ACTIONS
2 oz. ginkgo leaf *(Ginkgo biloba)*	Improves memory, mood, blood vessels
2 oz. eleuthero root *(Eleutherococcus senticosus)*	Strengthens stress response, immune resistance
3 oz. lemon balm leaf *(Melissa officinalis)*	For taste, digestion; lifts mood
1 oz. skullcap herb *(Scutellaria laterifolia)*	Relaxes tension; mildly calming
Optional, to taste: ¼ oz. ginger *(Zingiber officinale)*	Stimulates circulation to the brain

See the previous recipe for information about the mixture's benefits and length of use. Again, the most lasting benefits come after several weeks.

Add ½ ounce of the mixture to 3 cups of boiling water in a teapot or container with a well-fitting lid. Let stand for twenty minutes before straining. Even though most of these herbs are leaves, whereas the eleuthero is a root, its constituents are not hard to extract in a well-covered teapot after the allotted time. Drink 1 cup, hot or cold, twice a day. Because these herbs are lightweight and fluffy, you may find them easier to handle if you make a big batch once every three days and refrigerate it. Preparing the tea in quantity also allows you to drink more than 2 cups a day, which is perfectly fine. It's safe, and your body will tell you if you want more on some days. For three days of strong tea, pour 2 quarts of boiling water over 2 ounces of herbs; let the mixture sit, covered, for thirty minutes, then strain and drink as desired. You should enjoy the taste of this tea, so make it as strong or weak as you wish.

Eight ounces will last two to three weeks.

When you can't get a good night's sleep, it's hard to have a good day. Occasional use of herbs can provide temporary relief from sleeplessness or pain and avoid dependence on stronger drugs. The following formulas avoid the possibility of drug interaction, and when taken as directed are non-habit-forming.

Note that the formulas use valerian, which is not the herbal source for the prescription drug Valium. Biochemically speaking, they have nothing to do with each other. However, if you are being treated for depression or are sensitive to alcohol, ask your health-care provider if you may use the milder tea. Three points about using valerian: First, it is the best herb for bringing on sleepiness, but some people have the opposite reaction—the sedative alkaloids in the plant make them feel as if they've drunk too much coffee. If this happens, even once, leave out the valerian. Second, other drugs, whether prescription or recreational, have the potential to sensitize the nervous system, making it react unpredictably. Some women find that valerian works well from the first few nights on, but the better studies done on this strong-smelling root show that the best effects are after taking it at least four or five nights in a row. This formula also helps with tension headaches.

Concentrate for restorative sleep

CONCENTRATED HERB EXTRACT	ACTIONS
4 oz. passionflower herb (*Passiflora incarnata*)	Safely inhibits pain; lowers anxiety; helps you stay asleep
2 oz. skullcap herb (*Scutellaria laterifolia*)	Relaxes muscle tension; calming
2 oz. valerian root (*Valeriana officinalis*)	Helps you get to sleep

For a change from my usual recommendations in this book, don't combine these herbal extracts until you have tried the herbs without valerian, and on another night, a dose of the whole herbal formula to compare for yourself. Mix ½ teaspoon of passionflower plus ¼ teaspoon each of skullcap and valerian in ⅓ cup of water or juice (white grape juice helps counteract the peculiar smell and taste). Drink the mixture twice: about an hour before bedtime and again at bedtime; repeat the dose if needed for a third time if you awaken sleepless or in pain during the night. Valerian is a great muscle-relaxing herb.

If you sleep better with it in the mix, go ahead and combine all the extracts. Eight ounces will last one to two weeks depending on need.

If you find you have a jittery reaction to the mixture with valerian, leave it out. Combine the passionflower and skullcap, and take 1 teaspoon of the combination in ⅓ cup of liquid as needed.

For temporary pain relief during the day, use smaller amounts: up to ½ teaspoon every hour or two as needed. Undiagnosed pain or untreated insomnia that lasts longer than one to two weeks is your signal to check with a care provider.

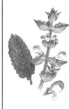

Tea for restorative sleep

DRIED HERBS

4 oz. passionflower herb *(Passiflora incarnata)*

2 oz. skullcap herb *(Scutellaria laterifolia)*

2 oz. valerian root *(Valeriana officinalis)*

ACTIONS

Safely inhibits pain; lowers anxiety; helps you stay asleep

Relaxes muscle tension; calming

Helps you get to sleep

This tea is not delicious, but it works for many women. Start by adding 1 ounce of the mixture to 2½ cups of boiling water in a teapot or container with a well-fitting lid. Let stand for fifteen minutes before straining. Drink 1 cup, hot or cold, an hour before bed; then drink ½ cup half an hour before bed, and, if needed, another ½ cup at bedtime. Remember to empty your bladder last thing before going to bed. You can sip another cup if pain or agitation awaken you during the night. During the day, drink ½ cup as needed for temporary pain relief. Any undiagnosed pain or untreated insomnia that lasts longer than one to two weeks is a signal for you to check with a care provider. Valerian may be omitted if you can't get past the taste or if you have any negative sensitivity to it.

Eight ounces will last two weeks depending on need.

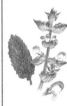

Concentrate and tea for optimal memory

CONCENTRATED HERB EXTRACT

1 oz. gotu kola *(Centella asiatica)*

1 oz. bacopa *(Bacopa monniera, sometimes B. monnieri)*

¼ oz. rosemary *(Rosmarinus officinalis)*

ACTIONS

Aids skin and nerve health

Nervine; improves mental performance, memory

Antioxidant; digestive and memory aid

Combine these extracts and take ½ teaspoon in water every morning.

Two and a quarter ounces will last about three weeks. You could also just take a tablet. Also known as brahmi, Bacopa monniera *products should state on the label that they deliver the equivalent of 3 grams dry weight with 60 percent bacosides.*

This exact formula can be made as a tea. Combine these leaves and steep 1 teaspoon in 1 cup water just off the boil. Steep for five to ten minutes; strain out the tea leaves. Drink 1 cup at least once a day or as often as you like. This is a caffeine-free approach to stimulating the nerves for mental function while providing antioxidants.

Nutrition

Review the following suggestions for whole foods that provide vitamins and minerals to address the nervous system, as well as the list of natural supplements.

wise food choices

❋ Eat a walnut every day, plain or broken and unheated, in vegetable or grain dishes. Walnuts and many other nuts provide a small amount of essential fatty acids, vegetable protein, vitamins B and E, calcium, iron, potassium, magnesium, and other nutrients. According to folklore, walnuts are associated with better brain power; one a day isn't enough to be fattening.

❋ Avoid eating dairy foods in excess. Cheese and butter, for example, are loaded with fat and salt, which clog arteries, affecting blood supply everywhere, including the brain.

❋ If you do not get indigestion from garlic, eat a raw or steamed clove every day to lower cholesterol, help general immunity, and improve circulation, necessary for getting oxygen to the brain.

supplements

❋ To add to memory and mental clarity, take gotu kola (*Centella asiatica*), a bitter-tasting tropical trailing vine available in tablets and as a liquid extract. Use as directed on labels. Gotu kola is also an excellent remedy for improving the health of skin, used externally and taken internally. I grow it as a houseplant and eat three fresh leaves a day.

❋ Bacopa (*Bacopa monniera*) is perhaps best known for its memory-enhancing benefits; it also is an antioxidant. Bacopa helps our livers in their detoxifying functions. This herb, called the scholar's herb because of its effects on clear thinking, also aids spleen function. The spleen is a big lymphatic storehouse, sheltering a reserve of red blood cells and infection-fighting white blood cells. The spleen is where old red blood cells get recycled and where the essence of nutrition is extracted for use as energy, after the small intestine and liver have their way with the foods we eat.

These self-cleansing functions of the body may explain why bacopa is traditionally used to treat skin conditions from acne and infection to eczema and psoriasis. Bacopa necessarily acts on a congested digestive tract, easing constipation through its liver-stimulating activity. As an all-around immune aid, bacopa is a relaxing expectorant, which means it is effective at quieting bronchitis, asthma, and coughs. Finally, because the role that stress plays in immune resistance is crucial, bacopa has an antianxiety effect that is not sedating and even increases energy.

In Addition

❋ Carry a small vial of essential oil of peppermint (available at any drugstore). Place a drop on a cotton ball and place it in the car or near your desk. In aromatherapy experiments, peppermint in factory air vents significantly increased alertness and improved mood.

* Grow a rosemary plant indoors or out. Eat one leaf each day, making sure you chew it slowly. Rub the fragrant leaves between your fingers while on the phone or reading something important. The next time you rub rosemary leaves or sniff its essential oil, your recall will be better.

* Exercise of any type that suits you improves every aspect of mental clarity. Even a slow, stately walk clears the mind, massages the heart, and draw forth hidden wellsprings of inspiration.

IMMUNE STRENGTH

Immune function does not automatically worsen because of age, but it may seem that way, especially if you are frequently exposed to children or the public and constantly get colds, flu, and other infections. The following formulas help rebuild your immunity to avoid colds, flus, common urinary-tract infections, and shingles. As we age, we tend to compromise on our nutrition—this may mean that we are also getting less protein, iron, and other important dietary factors that bolster immunity and prevent infection. If you are getting sick often, it is important to make sure you are getting all of your dietary nutrients. Insomnia can also compromise immunity—a lot of important reparative functions happen while we sleep, so if poor sleep and frequent colds or infections are going hand in hand in your life, sometimes treating the former can help with the latter.

Colds and Flu

As you age, you will have a special need to keep minor colds and flu from settling into your lungs to avoid the need for antibiotics or medical care for more serious problems. This is especially true if arthritis limits your chest expansion, when we may rely too heavily on upper back muscles expanding. You can alleviate minor conditions on your own; serious infections such as pneumonia require professional care. Most women can distinguish between a common problem and an uncommon medical need, but when common sense causes you to feel doubt, check with a professional.

The following formula, taken either as a combination of extracts or as a tea, can help prevent early signs of illness, especially to keep sore throats and colds from settling in the chest, and it can help fight off an already-established infection. It provides a whole-body immune tune-up that covers sinus, lung, throat, stomach, intestinal, and lymph node infections that are not life threatening. This can be taken along with or after antibiotics, without negative interaction. Many people may think of echinacea first for any infection, but it isn't necessary to use it every time, and it isn't the best at fighting colds or flu, which is why it is at the bottom of the list for this type of immune system therapy. Include echinacea in the combination only when infections are stubborn or repeated more than twice in a winter.

Herbal Medicine

Concentrate for colds and flu

CONCENTRATED HERB EXTRACT

3 oz. mint leaf *(Mentha* species*)*

2 oz. sage leaf *(Salvia officinalis)*

1 oz. rosemary herb *(Rosmarinus officinalis)*

1 oz. black cohosh root *(Cimicifuga racemosa)*

1 oz. elderberry *(Sambucus nigra)*

ANY OR ALL OF THE FOLLOWING MAY BE USED OPTIONALLY; VARY AMOUNTS TO TASTE:

¼ oz. licorice root *(Glycyrrhiza glabra)*

¼ oz. ginger root *(Zingiber officinale)*

1 oz. echinacea root *(Echinacea* species*)*

ACTIONS

Disguises flavor; aids digestion of remedy

Relieves sore throats; antiseptic; cleansing

Antiseptic for sinus, lungs, stomach

For muscle stiffness, congested lungs from flu

For antiviral effects

Antiviral; soothing for dry coughs

Warming for a cold; settles the stomach

Broad-spectrum antimicrobial; immune aid for more stubborn infections

Combine these herbal extracts. Take 1 teaspoon in 1 cup of water, juice, or any herb tea every hour for the first day or two; then continue, even if feeling better, four times a day, tapering off to twice a day, morning and evening, until two to three weeks are up.

Eight ounces without the optional additions, or up to 9 ounces including any or all of those, will last two to three weeks.

Nutrition

Review the following suggestions for whole foods that provide vitamins and minerals to address immune system health, as well as the list of natural supplements.

wise food choices

❀ Add a pinch of thyme to broth, soups, or cooked grains daily for three days.

❀ Add 1 ounce dried or 3 ounces fresh shiitake mushrooms every other day to cooked foods, stir-fried vegetable dishes, soups, broths, and casseroles. These delicious mushrooms are available dried or fresh in Asian produce sections of grocery stores; like many specialized or wild mushrooms, they build nonspecific immunity.

❀ Add a pinch of cayenne (red pepper) to foods for vitamin C and antimicrobial volatile oils to protect against colds. Some hearty older women sprinkle it on salads or brown rice; others stir ¼ teaspoon into a glass of water at room temperature and knock it back as a daily winter preventative. If cayenne disagrees with your constitution, as with any food or herb, don't force yourself to use it.

❀ Turmeric, the yellow herb in curry powder blends, is an antioxidant and immune booster. Enjoy frequent curry dishes, adding it according to taste.

supplements

❀ Vitamin C with bioflavonoids from food sources (for example, acerola), 2 to 6 grams per day for ten days. Excess vitamin C may cause looseness of stool; if this occurs, reduce or drop the dose to bowel tolerance.

❀ Grape seed extract, taken as directed on labels. An excellent antioxidant, grape seed has several immune benefits.

In Addition

❀ A cold is just that—a drop in your temperature. A normal body temperature of 98.6°F or so kills off normal populations of unwanted germs that we encounter as part of everyday life. When these common microbes build up to levels that our first defenses cannot manage, a raised body temperature is nature's way of cooking the germs. Though this simple approach is not for every infection, whatever the temperature, the familiar common cold responds to getting ourselves warmed up, but with common sense. Soak your body in a comfortably hot bath for at least twenty minutes. In the process, you will also be sweating out impurities, lessening the burden on your immune system. Optionally, you may add five to ten drops of one or more of your favorite disinfecting and mood-sweetening essential oils: rose (expensive, but a few drops are a powerful and safe disinfectant for all skin types), sandalwood, cedarwood, aniseed, birch, sage, rosemary. Use only two to four drops of the following stronger oils: lemon, eucalyptus, ti tree, (also known as tea tree [*Melaleuca alternifolia, M. quinquenervia*]).

❀ If you don't have a bathtub or if you prefer showers, add these essential oils to shower gels or place drops in the corners of the shower stall and turn the water to very hot for a volatile, cleansing, steamy shower.

❀ Try this visualization: Drink a cup of herb tea, then sit back in your hot bath or in bed. Imagine ("image in") your white blood cells receiving magic droplets of botanical biochemicals, equipping them to rove out into every place in your body that is tender or hot. See the outsiders—viruses, fungi, and bacteria—stopping in their tracks as your immune cells explain that they must move elsewhere. Subdued and repenting any harm they may have caused, the microbes let their weakened forces be swept into the lymph nodes for neutralizing and from there to pathways of excretion for a speedy exit. Recycled as pieces of harmless matter, they are restored to the vast pool of a living Earth to find their rightful spot.

Urinary-Tract Infections

When prescriptions and creams don't work, the following herb formulas can help your own defenses combat cystitis and other common urinary-tract infections. Cystitis is an inflammation of the bladder that usually but not always occurs with an infection. But there is an exception: interstitial cystitis (IC) feels like a urinary-tract infection, but there are no bacteria in the urine. Some doctors believe that in some cases of IC infections actually do occur, but with organisms like chlamydia, which are not usually looked for when cystitis symptoms appear. On the other hand, antibiotics have been considered as one possible cause of IC, as an allergic type of response. The pain of IC is worse as the bladder fills, so frequent trips to the bathroom are perhaps annoying but advisable. The long-term nature of the problem may not respond quickly to the following herbs, but the formulas will at least help flush an increased fluid volume through the urinary tract to prevent secondary infections, spasm, and pain.

The following formulas are designed with the older woman in mind, so they are different from the formulas for cystitis included in chapter 2. Note that a bladder infection (cystitis) and stress incontinence (weak bladder tone) are not the same, but the following herbal approach will help in either case.

Herbal Medicine

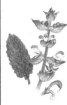

Concentrate for urinary-tract health

CONCENTRATED HERB EXTRACT

2 oz. marshmallow root *(Althaea officinalis)*

2 oz. cramp bark *(Viburnum opulus)*

2 oz. bearberry leaf *(Arctostaphylos uva-ursi)*

ACTIONS

Coats and protects vulnerable tissue linings; soothing diuretic

Relaxes spasms; allows urinary stream to flow

Disinfects; stimulates urine flow

Combine these herbal extracts. Take 1 teaspoon to 1 tablespoon in 1 cup of water, juice, or any herb tea every hour for one day. Follow with 1 teaspoon in water twice a day until symptoms subside. If any infection does not respond in two days, see your health-care provider. If microbes are still present, continue using the remedy for another two weeks, with monitoring by your health-care provider. These herbs work with or without antibiotics. For IC, add to either the extract or the tea 1 ounce nettle leaf (Urtica dioica), *1 ounce echinacea root (any* Echinacea *species), and 2 ounces St. John's wort herb* (Hypericum perforatum), *also a fine liver and immune herb.*

    Six ounces will last about one week.

Tea for urinary-tract health

DRIED HERBS

3 oz. marshmallow root *(Althaea officinalis)*

3 oz. bearberry leaf *(Arctostaphylos uva-ursi)*

2 oz. cramp bark *(Viburnum opulus)*

ACTIONS

Coats and protects vulnerable tissue linings; soothing diuretic

Disinfects; stimulates urine flow

Relaxes spasms; allows urinary stream to flow

Add 1 ounce to 3½ cups of boiling water in a teapot or container with a well-fitting lid. Let stand for fifteen minutes before straining. Drink 1 cup, at room temperature or cold, three times a day until symptoms subside. If the infection does not respond in two days, see your health-care provider. Continue drinking the tea for another week even if antibiotics are needed.

    Eight ounces will last about two weeks.

Shingles

Shingles is caused by a member of the herpes family of viruses, *Herpes zoster*, that stays dormant in the nerve cells. When it flares up, it causes a painful skin outbreak, usually in a single continuous patch or line. It flares up during periods of depressed immunity, including depression and emotional strain, and is a problem in all immunocompromised people who have ever had chicken pox. Chronic shingles especially flares up after medical procedures or other stressful experiences. When the virus damages a nerve that supplies the skin with sensation, the sensation on the skin is searing pain, while the skin may remain normal or may break out in raised red bumps. If scratched, the rash may itch, bleed, or become infected, and it may be too painful to be covered with clothing or a bedsheet. When it is possible to use remedies on the surface, such as at the very first warning sign, tingling pain, you can apply external remedies to the skin (see "In Addition").

The conventional medical treatment is with antiviral drugs and pain relievers. Although no herb is known to eliminate shingles or other herpes infections entirely, several studies back up the claim that garlic and other inexpensive natural remedies are effective. The following formula contains antiviral herbs that restore strength and immune resistance to the nerve tissues. You can take it for a few weeks or even a few months at a time for prevention as well as treatment during outbreaks. Any shingles infection that does not respond in ten days requires professional care, as does shingles that occurs on the face, especially near the eyes. Most people head for help long before ten days.

If you have high blood pressure or a weak heart or kidneys, replace licorice root with an equal amount of golden root (*Rhodiola rosea*) or eleuthero (*Eleutherococcus senticosus*). Both have immunity-building and stress-reducing properties yet do not have the overstimulation side effects sometimes seen with Korean or Chinese ginseng.

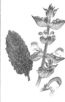

Concentrate for reducing episodes of shingles

CONCENTRATED HERB EXTRACT	ACTIONS
2 oz. St. John's wort herb (*Hypericum perforatum*)	Antiviral; repairs nerves; anti-inflammatory
1 oz. licorice root (*Glycyrrhiza glabra*)	Antiviral; anti-inflammatory; harmonizes
2 oz. echinacea root (*Echinacea purpurea*)	Antiviral; reduces risk of secondary infection
1 oz. kanuka (*Kunzea ericoides*)	New Zealand native antiviral, antifungal; if unavailable, increase echinacea to a total of 3 oz.
2 oz. eleuthero root (*Eleutherococcus senticosus*)	Improves effect of echinacea and other antiviral herbs

Combine the tinctures and store in a dark glass bottle with a label and a tight-fitting lid. Take ½ to 1 teaspoon (2.5 to 5 milliliters) three times a day for ten days. You may want to chase it with pear juice, which has antiviral properties.

Alternatively, this can be mixed as powdered dried herbs, 2 #00 capsules taken three times a day for two weeks.

Eight ounces will last about two weeks.

Nutrition

Review the following suggestions for whole foods that provide vitamins and minerals to address immune resistance and repair.

wise food choices

❀ Garlic is the primary antagonist of the *H. zoster* virus that causes shingles. Garlic can be taken as deodorized garlic perles, 1000 milligrams per day for ten days or while an outbreak threatens. Allicin is the constituent that has been thought most important, though now a complex of constituents are believed to be bioactive. Raw or lightly steamed garlic seems to have more immune-fighting power than cooked or deodorized products do. Aim for three cloves per day, pressed onto freshly buttered toast, tossed over salad, or disguised in 1 tablespoon of raw, local, unheated honey. Propolis and bee pollen also have antiviral properties.

❀ The amino acid lysine, found in many foods, is an essential amino acid (meaning we cannot make it in the body). Lysine is protective against herpes, as it is needed for immune resistance and repair, along with other functions. It is believed that lysine, which is similar in shape to the herpes virus, is absorbed into the virus. On the other hand, the amino acid arginine, though it offers other health benefits, is associated with outbreaks because the virus feeds on arginine. Two confirmed triggers for herpes outbreaks besides high stress are eating a diet high in arginine-rich foods and/or consuming a diet that leads to a lysine deficiency. Some arginine-containing food can be eaten in moderation by those with a history of herpes when they are in good health otherwise. Other people find that avoiding the riskier arginine foods as a general rule is the best prevention. The first list below is of foods high in lysine, which are helpful to emphasize in the diet regularly, to your taste. Although clinical lysine deficiency is uncommon in North America and many industrialized countries, lysine is destroyed by cooking foods at very high temperatures. This list of helpful foods is followed by "trigger" foods high in arginine, which should be avoided in excess or during periods of illness and stress.

HIGH-LYSINE FOODS TO EMPHASIZE

* Fresh fish
* Canned fish
* Chicken
* Goat's milk
* Cooked mung beans
* Cooked beans, various
* Fresh watercress
* Cooked black beans, lentils, or soy
* Star fruit
* Papaya
* Grapefruit, apricot, pear, apple, fig

HIGH-ARGININE FOODS TO LIMIT OR AVOID

* Hazelnuts
* Brazil nuts
* Peanuts
* Walnuts
* Almond
* Cocoa powder
* Peanut butter
* Sesame seeds
* Brown rice

supplements

* Lysine: 500 to 2000 milligrams a day for thirty days; 500 milligrams a day for maintenance. Lysine creams may be helpful externally.

* Vitamin A, vitamin C, and zinc in combination improve the function of the immune system. Take in a food-source multivitamin at double the recommended dose for five days only.

* Beta 1,3 glucan is an immune-building starch (immunomodulating polysaccharide) found in shiitake and other medicinal, edible mushrooms. Follow label directions on standardized extracts during outbreaks. Eat two mushrooms in food every day as a maintenance dose.

* Resveratrol, found in grape seed, red wine, and chocolate, may prevent the herpes virus from replicating in human cells. The benefits of these foods may lead you to eat them unless the arginine in chocolate is not balanced by eating other foods rich in lysine, or if there is a reason to avoid red wine, as in the discussion regarding some types of arthritic joint pain.

In Addition

* Apply the following external herb oil for temporary pain numbing and antiviral and anti-itch properties. Combine in a bottle with a spray top: 1 ounce St. John's wort oil (available at herb shops or from the businesses in Resources) and ¼ ounce essential oil of peppermint (available at many drugstores as well as aromatherapy and herb companies); for added strength, you can add the pressed juice of two garlic cloves. Store in the refrigerator for up to six months. Shake well before each spray application of herbal mist.

  Because the oils eventually break down the plastic, store in glass until needed. Glass bottles with sprayers are preferable, but recycled, sterilized plastic bottles can be used. Spray a light mist on painful skin as needed. It doesn't have to be rubbed in, but be aware that it will stain clothing and it smells strongly of mint (and garlic if added).

VAGINAL CHANGES

More than ever before, postmenopausal women are seeking information on how to keep their sex life thriving as they age. Many women are even beginning relationships in this new life stage, so a new love in your sixties or later shouldn't surprise anyone. There's no mystery to having good sex during this stage of life. In health, humans can enjoy sex as long as they keep the pump primed. When age-related problems get in the way of your enjoyment, acceptance of the situation, taking your time, and using herbal remedies can make all the difference.

Among postmenopausal women, two primary obstacles to good sex are vaginal dryness and atrophy. *Atrophy* means "lack of growth" but can really mean thinning vaginal walls or loss of cushioning fat. If the pain you feel with sex seems to be from vaginal dryness, see the discussion and remedies in chapter 2. Vaginal atrophy is commonly used to mean drying, thinning, and shrinking of the vaginal wall. An inflammatory condition related to less estrogen and thus, less lubrication, atrophy can make the lining of the vagina less flexible and vulnerable to tearing. Atrophy also includes a generalized loss of tone in the connective tissues of the pelvis, causing the organs contained in the pelvis to drop (prolapse).

Postmenopausal atrophy may take up to ten years to show up and is more than simple vaginal dryness. After menopause, the labia minora (Latin for "little lips," the folds of skin enclosing the vaginal opening) may disappear, while the labia majora (the larger, outer pair of vaginal lips) become thinner. The vagina itself becomes smaller, the lining thinner and less "tough." As a result, irritations and infections may become chronic and immune defense less abundant, especially if circulation and nutrition are poor. The supportive ligaments of the pelvis lose some of their tone, making the organs they support more vulnerable to prolapse (dropping down out of place). Moreover, starting at the onset of menopause, the cervix slowly decreases in size, and the secretory glands it contains may become less active with less sexual stimulation. Because the uterine lining stops thickening and shedding in a monthly cycle, and the uterus knows it won't have to push another infant into the world now, the muscle layer of the uterus thins. But not to worry: this change is not problematic as long as you take care to maintain health and guard against minor infections, abrasions, inflammations, and dry spells—conditions that our vaginas could recover from more easily fifteen years ago but are now more likely to get our full attention.

Maintaining natural lubrication protects you from infections caused by microbes, even sneaky ones that can exploit a lack of immunity at this doorway to the body, traveling up the urethral opening close to the vagina and possibly leading to bladder infections (see the section on urinary-tract infections earlier in this chapter). Because these vaginal infections involve both the reproductive and the urinary tracts, the natural methods for preventing or treating them utilize herbs with an affinity for both body systems. It is a revelation to study the qualities of such doubly helpful herbs, only to realize that some of them are hormonal-normalizing tonics as well. Nature has provided for women in every bioregion. Herbal or "all natural" sexual lubricants and stimulants are a big business; although new products are worth investigating, that doesn't mean all are worth buying. We're looking for research on safety as well as effectiveness, as scores of new products hit the marketplace every year.

The use of the following tea over three to six months improves vaginal tissue health. This happens in part by preventing infections caused by dryness, even though vaginal walls may be thinner. The herbs cannot guarantee a lack of infection but can add gentle anti-inflammatory and healing properties to the skin's natural immune defenses. The tea can be used in addition to, or after short-term use of, the extract below.

Herbal Medicine

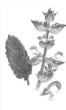

Concentrate for improved intimacy

CONCENTRATED HERB EXTRACT	ACTIONS
2 oz. ashwagandha *(Withania somniferum)*	Adaptogen; restorative tonic
2 oz. shatavari *(Asparagus racemosa)*	Moistening; aids libido
1 oz. damiana herb *(Turnera diffusa)*	Nervine tonic for energy and circulation to genitalia
1 oz. dong quai root *(Angelica sinensis)*	Optimizes healthy flow of blood
2 oz. ginseng root *(Panax* species)	Increases endurance; lessens fatigue; supports long-term immunity and sexual vitality

Panax *ginseng is Chinese or Korean ginseng, usually cured to a red color; it is more heating than white roots of American ginseng* (Panax quinquefolium). *Both are excellent adaptogens as well as aids to stamina and longevity. The more heating Chinese ginseng is contraindicated for women with high blood pressure, headaches, or insomnia, or those using caffeine or some prescribed medications. Use American ginseng in those cases, and always take note of your own sensitivity to stimulating herbs.*

Combine these herbal extracts. Take 1 teaspoon in 1 cup of water, juice, or any herb tea three times a day for at least two weeks. Best results are seen in three to four weeks.

Note: *If you experience any spotting postmenopausally or note blood in the urine, consult your health-care provider; meanwhile, discontinue this extract combination. Replace with 2 ounces fresh plant extract of shepherd's purse* (Capsella bursa-pastoris) *combined with 2 ounces echinacea extract* (Echinacea *species): take 1 teaspoon diluted in anything to get it down, four times a day for a minimum of three days, even if spotting improves. Don't neglect obtaining a medical diagnosis even if these two herbs seem to clear this symptom.*

Eight ounces will last two weeks to thirty days.

Tea for improved intimacy

DRIED HERBS	ACTIONS
1 oz. raspberry leaf (*Rubus idaeus*)	As tea, delicate source of isoflavones with estrogen-like effect on tissue; astringent tonic; mild diuretic
2 oz. fennel seeds (*Foeniculum vulgare*)	Provides phytoestrogens; for taste
3 oz. damiana herb (*Turnera diffusa*)	Nervine tonic for energy and genitalia
2 oz. peppermint leaf (*Mentha piperita*)	For taste; digestion of other herbs

Add ¼ ounce of the mixture to 3 cups of boiling water in a teapot or container with a well-fitting lid. Let stand for ten to fifteen minutes before straining. Drink 1 cup, hot or cold, two to three times a day for at least two weeks. Repeat as often or as long as you like. Can be enjoyed by either gender. If taken longer than three months, skip one or two days per week.

Eight ounces will last about thirty days.

Nutrition

Review the following suggestions for whole foods that provide vitamins and minerals to address vaginal changes.

wise food choices

❀ Omega-3 essential fatty acids are essential to lubrication and repair of many tissues.

❀ Eat soybeans and fermented soy foods for increased lubrication and fiber. Soy is not only heart-healthy, but the fiber is also beneficial for everything from blood sugar to sex hormones. And soy is not the only, or even the best, source of phytoestrogens. Cook the widest variety of legumes (lentils, peas, beans) with epazote, fennel, celery seeds, cilantro, and other aromatic culinary herbs that you like, to improve their digestibility.

❀ See also the recommendations under "Vaginal Thinning and Dryness" in chapter 2. You can use the same nutritional recommendations and external remedies for postmenopausal dryness and thinning.

In Addition

❀ Massage five drops of essential oil of chaste berry (*Vitex agnus-castus*) into the abdomen daily. Many women who do this experience increased vaginal lubrication in just one week.

The jury is still deliberating on whether local estrogen for vaginal changes (for example, the Estring, estrogen creams, or tablets) are as safe as previously believed.

❀ Zestra is an over-the-counter product that contains borage seed oil, evening primrose oil, angelica root extract, *Coleus forskohlii* extract, vitamin C, and vitamin E. It is applied to the clitoris five minutes before sex to improve sensation. It has been shown in a small but well-designed trial to be safe and effective, both before and after menopause, and may even decrease the side effect some antidepressants (SSRIs) have of reducing sex drive.

❀ Vibrel, widely advertised, is a gel containing niacin, a natural vasodilator, to increase circulation to women's reproductive tissues, with a resulting increase in pleasure.

❀ Emerita is a line of natural lubricants that are water-based (latex friendly), paraben-free, and supportive of menopausal women's vaginal health and pleasure.

appendix a
Guidelines for Preparing Herbs

CONCENTRATES, EXTRACTS, AND TINCTURES

These terms are not precisely interchangeable, but in this book, for the sake of simplicity, I have used the term *concentrates* to mean concentrated extracts. Also called *tinctures*, these concentrated herbal preparations last indefinitely, unlike teas, and can be taken in small amounts. Five to ten drops of tincture diluted in a little water may be the most effective way to take a remedy, not to mention that this is more convenient than brewing up a pot of tea. Some women find that 1 teaspoon of tincture, either a formula or a single herb extract, that is diluted in a little juice, herb tea, or water, does the trick in twenty minutes. This is often repeated two or three times in a day, for a therapeutic herbal dose on average of 3 teaspoons a day. On the other hand, a tea may take longer—twenty minutes to an hour to feel the benefits.

Not all active chemical constituents in herbs are water-soluble, so alcohol or another solvent is usually necessary to fully extract the herb's properties. Vegetable glycerin is a commonly used solvent; even vinegar can be an effective solvent for some herbs. Tinctures in alcohol bases are the most commonly available commercially, and the amount of alcohol per dose is relatively small. If, however, you are unable to use alcohol-based herb preparations, you can readily replace them with glycerin-based or other nonalcohol-based extracts, herb teas, aromatherapy, and even herb oils for absorption through the skin. A common belief is that adding boiling water to alcohol tinctures burns off the alcohol, and this helps, but some alcohol is left afterward, and some heat-sensitive herb properties may be lost.

Dosage varies from an average of 3 teaspoons per day (15 milliliters), depending on who is taking it. A general guideline is to use ½ to 1 teaspoon in ½ to 1 cup of water three times a day. Small or sensitive women may start with ½ teaspoon; those with strong constitutions or more demanding health concerns find that a beginning dose of 1 teaspoon is more effective. Glycerin tinctures are usually less potent than alcohol tinctures, so you can take a little more.

Tinctures are expensive in retail herb shops and many online suppliers. To be sure you are getting high quality as well as reasonable prices, see my favorite companies, listed in the Resources. You may also want to make your own. Concentrated extracts or tinctures are easier to make than many people think. In the doses recommended in this book, they are often more effective and far more affordable than some retail products. Here is how it is done: Whether you are using one herb or a combination, place 5 ounces in a blender or food processor and shred the material into small pieces (but it needn't be a powder), then put it into a glass jar or other container with a tight lid. Add 25 ounces of at least 40-percent alcohol (80 proof or stronger, such as medium-priced brandy or vodka). Store out of direct light and away from heat sources (a convenient spot in your kitchen cupboard, for instance). Once every day for fourteen days, shake the closed container to evenly mix the liquid and herb pieces. After two weeks, strain the mixture through a piece of clean muslin large enough that you can wrap it up and squeeze out the last few drops of liquid. Store the extract in a dark glass bottle with a lid (a brown bottle from your drugstore or a sterilized green wine bottle with a cork). Label the container clearly with the date, the name of the herb, the name of the person it is for, and the dose.

Tinctures do not require refrigeration; store, capped tightly, away from direct heat, light, and children.

TEAS

Herbal teas can be steeped (infused) or simmered (decocted).

Infusions

Leaves, flowers, and delicate parts of plants with fragrance are best steeped, 1 ounce of dried herb to three 8-ounce cups of just-boiled water. Put the herb in a teapot or nonmetal container, pour the water over the herb, and cover with a well-fitting lid. Allow the tea to sit, or steep, for five to twenty-five minutes, usually about fifteen, before straining out the herb and discarding it. Drink from ½ to 1 cup of tea two or three times a day. As a general guideline for herb teas in this book, 1 teaspoon is loosely equivalent to 2 grams, but this is sometimes inexact because of variation in herb density; therefore, recipes usually specify weights, such as 1 ounce to a pint.

Decoctions

Place the tough parts of herbs, such as roots, bark, seeds, and berries, in cold water, 1 ounce of dried herb to 3 cups of water, in a stainless steel or other suitable vessel covered with a well-fitting lid. Bring the pot to a simmer over low heat and leave it at the lowest possible heat for five to twenty-five minutes, usually fifteen, before straining out the herb and discarding it. Take ½ to 1 cup of tea two to three times a day.

Many herb combinations contain both leaves and flowers as well as roots and seeds. If you have the time, you can separately simmer the roots, bark, berries, and seeds in the total amount of water and for the same period called for, then turn off the heat and add the leaves, flowers, and herbs, and let them steep for the usual fifteen minutes or the specified time before straining. Seeds or other materials that have a strong aroma because they contain volatile oils should be added at the steeping step. This method results in the strongest combinations. If you are short on time, the combinations in this book will work just fine if you prepare the herbs all at once; just let the roots and leaves sit, or steep, an extra few minutes. Combinations using extracts do not require any special preparation: each root or flower has already been extracted, so you just combine them and take as directed.

Sweeten teas with a little honey if you wish, but do not use refined sugar. You can make enough tea to last three days, store it in the refrigerator, and drink it hot or cold or at room temperature; you can also reheat a cup at a time. Herb tea will not last longer than three days, even covered and refrigerated.

How long should you take these teas? No book can pretend to know exactly for each woman's case, but as a guide, acute problems should respond in a few doses or a few days. These are best treated with a dose every ten to twenty minutes or at least every one to two hours as needed until you feel better. Then take one dose two to three times a day for another few days. In cases of infection, continue taking herbs for seven to ten days past the acute stage to help the body's recovery and prevent recurrence.

Chronic conditions should show some sign of improvement in one to three weeks even if all symptoms do not respond at once. For the best outcome, take herbs three times a day for at least one to three months, in some cases up to a year for permanent improvement.

EXTERNAL PREPARATIONS: HERB OILS AND SALVES

Many herbs—such as wild yam, comfrey, calendula, and St. John's wort—can be extracted in oil and then applied externally or vaginally daily and during intercourse for lubrication. Or you can add essential oils like lavender, clary sage, and jasmine to them and use them as massage and bath oils.

To make an herb oil, place 4 ounces of dried herb in a clean, dry quart jar, shake the herbs to settle them, and add green unfiltered olive oil, sesame oil, or almond oil to 1 inch above the level of herb in the container. Cover with a well-fitting but *not* completely tightened lid, and leave the jar in a constantly warm place (top of the refrigerator or water heater) for ten days.

At the end of this time, strain out the herb material and discard it, in your garden compost if possible. What remains is herb oil. Store away from sunlight and heat, preferably in a dark bottle with a well-fitting lid. Label it clearly and use within one year. If the oil begins to smell "off," it is contaminated and should be discarded.

If you can't wait ten days, follow these directions: Screw on the lid, but don't fully tighten it, and place the jar upright in a pan of water or double boiler over low heat for four hours. When the oil has the color and aroma of the herb, strain it through a fine filter, cheesecloth, or unbleached muslin. Avoid overheating, or the finished herb oil will smell burnt, even rancid—not an incentive to use it.

If you want to turn herb oil into a salve, do the following: Return the oil to a clean, dry saucepan. Add 1 tablespoon of coconut butter or cocoa butter per ¼ cup of oil, and warm the mixture over low heat until dissolved. Pour into a clean, dry jar with a well-fitting lid, and label. If the combination is too soupy for convenient vaginal application, add more coconut or cocoa butter, or reheat the mixture and melt in one or more walnut-size pieces of beeswax to adjust the solidity of the salve. To test the consistency until it's right, dip a spoon into the mixture, place the spoon in the refrigerator for five minutes, then check the hardness of the salve. The salve's consistency does not lessen the therapeutic benefits of the herb oil, so prepare it according to your individual preference. Whenever you handle salve, use a teaspoon, not your fingers, to minimize contamination.

Some herb salves are multipurpose, but note that any oil-based preparation is not ideal when yeast or fungal infections are present because these life forms thrive in moist, hot environments, and salves help keep warmth and moisture in tissues. In these situations, use herb tinctures or extracts, because the alcohol helps dry the fungal infection.

St. John's wort oil should be a red color; it acts as an anti-inflammatory lubricant. Calendula oil should be golden; it is especially good for healing small tears or abrasions in vaginal mucosa. Both are antiviral, though the extent of their effectiveness is variable. Wild yam oil is the basis for many natural creams used specifically in menopause because it improves vaginal lubrication and reduces inflammation. In addition, its plant sterols may be absorbed, promoting local tissue changes or systemic health effects. It is not proven that wild yam salves promote hormonal balance (though the herb taken as tea or extract does have proven hormonal effects on stress and inflammation, at least). Comfrey carries no warnings or cautions when used vaginally for moistening dry mucous membranes; in fact, nothing is better for thin, inflamed, or raw surfaces.

How to Make Your Own Menopause Formula

If you would like to create an herbal formula that addresses your particular menopause health concerns, the following guidelines can help you make sense of the kaleidoscope of healing plants from which to choose.

IDENTIFYING HEALTH CHALLENGES

❀ If possible, ask older female relatives, especially your mother, about their own experiences with menopause. See if you can discern any patterns in your family's history. Some evidence from research suggests that family history is not important, though many women who have asked within the circles of female relatives would argue that more information is always worth having.

❀ List your most important health challenges.

Sadly, many of the mothers, older aunts, and even grandmothers of women entering menopause today had hysterectomies at an early age, so there is no natural history of menopause from which to learn. Even if that is true in your family, take a quiet ten minutes to write your most important health challenges on a sheet of paper. Identify your single most important concern. Try to be concise; describe your top priority in a few words ("crippling hot flashes" or "risk of osteoporosis").

As you rate the seriousness of your health concerns, be honest with yourself. Your list is just for your eyes, for your judgment, for your health. For example: "Hot flashes are making me crazy; my mood swings would sort out if I could just get some sleep." Identifying sleep as a priority will help you decide which herbs to choose at the next stage of creating your personal formula.

Or, perhaps, "Hot flashes? Not a problem. Only had night sweats twice all year, after late-night coffee and great Mexican food. Eat right most of the time; no risk factors other than normal aging—no deep worries about my heart. Irregular cycle is a major problem—might get pregnant in my new relationship, and that would be hard on me." The major challenge here is to regulate menstrual cycles.

SETTING HEALTH GOALS

To get a complete picture of your state of health, compare your list of challenges to the items listed in the accompanying sidebar ("Seven Overlapping Areas of Concern for Menopausal Women"). Which items are on both lists? Those are the ones that probably need the most attention. After you identify what bothers you most, restate your problems as goals—the positive state of health you wish to achieve.

Redefining problems as positive goals is the best way to find out what you really want for yourself. For example, the problem of irritability might be expressed as a deep desire for tranquility. On a practical level, this step helps you recognize the health properties, or actions, of herbs that will take you where you want to go.

CHOOSING HERBS

Jot down one or two possible herbs for each of your most important areas of concern. While reading this book, have certain herbs seemed appropriate for meeting your needs? If so, list them in the appropriate category. If an herb appears more than once, it is probably a "keeper" for your customized formula.

Here are some guidelines for choosing herbs:

❀ Name just five to seven herbs, each with the greatest "bouquet" of herbal properties or actions you want. Concentrate on those meeting your greatest concern and needs.

❀ Check the dosage levels of your choices; note suggested combinations and cautions listed in the pages where the herbs you choose are mentioned.

❀ When in doubt, use smaller proportions of strong-tasting herbs.

❀ Put one herb with the largest number of actions that are important to you at the top of your list; use more of it compared with the others.

Your most important herb will probably be a tonic, which can be used safely long term and in liberal amounts. Strong herbs are meant to be used in small doses.

Herbs are not drugs. With common sense and the guidelines in this book, you can trust your intuition. Write out a list of your major complaints and the body system(s) in need of herbal support. Compare your list with the one that follows.

seven overlapping areas of concern for menopausal women

1. Hot flashes (cardiovascular system)

2. Osteoporosis (musculoskeletal system)

3. Vaginal dryness or atrophy, which may lead to increased incidence of cystitis (reproductive and urinary systems)

4. Irregular cycle and spotting (reproductive system)

5. Increased cardiovascular risk in proportion to low estrogen (reproductive and cardiovascular systems)

6. Pain and dysmenorrhea with characteristic "dragging" sensations (nervous and reproductive systems)

7. Links between arthritic changes with age, pain threshold, and depression (nervous system and musculoskeletal system)

Let's say you have listed all the herbs that meet your special concerns. This is not yet a formula. In fact, your list may include more than seven herbs, and all your body systems may seem to need help! Take a deep breath and relax. If you leave all the herbs on your long list in the final formula because they sound *soooo* nice, you may not see a clear benefit in your health. Narrow down the list to one nutritive tonic that can help more than one body system. Keep one herb for emotional equilibrium. Choose only *one* specific herb to answer your body's most urgent symptoms. Use at least 2 ounces of this main herb, and 1 ounce of each of the four to six "helper" herbs. You may, of course, have fewer than five to seven herbs in your formula.

If you have selected more than two or three herbs, consider your choices in light of three criteria: your constitution, nutrition, and state of mind. This approach, as explained in the next section, was first described by herbalist Billie Potts in her book *Witches Heal*.

Constitution: Choose the preventive herbs that will do the most good today and tomorrow. Which chronic problems need help? Pick the herbs with an affinity for toning the body system where these chronic problems occur. You can pick tonic herbs that also have specific benefit for menopausal issues. When we build up health in weak areas, our self-healing capacity can focus on the main one. In this way, we may use digestive tonics, even if nothing terribly "wrong" is occurring in the digestive system at the time. Herbs treat what is right as well as what is wrong, to make a stronger whole woman.

Nutrition: Which nourishing herbs will support the primary herb in other body systems? In answering this question, keep two factors in mind. First, your helper herbs will work even better if they are also known to help the primary symptom causing distress. For example, motherwort reduces the primary symptom of hot flashes, and it helps nourish the nerves, liver, and reproductive system as a whole, plus it can lower high blood pressure. Second, avoid use of exotic or expensive herbs grown remotely, and try to choose herbs that both meet your needs and are available in your local environment. By doing so, you support your own bioregion and local growers. Obtaining our nutrition locally enriches the global plant community, making the planet that much more whole.

State of mind: Choose an herb that reduces stress and relaxes muscles, which in turn may help circulation. The nervines tone or improve the nerves, antispasmodics relax muscles, and analgesics or anodynes relieve pain. This group of herbs includes skullcap, passionflower, wild oats, motherwort, and valerian.

PREPARING THE FINAL MIX

If you haven't already chosen a general reproductive tonic, consider these examples: raspberry leaf (*Rubus idaeus*), yarrow (*Achillea millefolium*), and lady's mantle (*Alchemilla vulgaris*). Does your formula need one or more of these in addition to the others you have selected? If one herb helps all the areas, great. If one herb covers two out of three health concerns, good job. If you just love a few herbs because of earlier experience with them or their descriptions ring a bell, go with them. Now you're ready to combine your choices.

Mix the hard pieces (roots, bark, seeds, berries) in a paper bag or bowl. In a separate container, combine all the lighter pieces (flowers, leaves, powders). If any of the "hard" herbs work by virtue of their smell (valerian root, cinnamon bark, fennel seeds), add them to the light herb material, first breaking up any large pieces.

Steep, or infuse, the light herbs in just-boiled water, covered with a lid, for five to thirty minutes. The longer they sit, the stronger they get. More than a half hour is not helpful, though, because volatile properties evaporate away and bitters and tannins intensify.

The harder herbs don't give up their medicinal properties so easily. Simmer bark, roots, and other dense herb bits in water for ten to forty-five minutes (an average of twenty minutes), covered with a lid.

If you wish, you can first simmer the hard pieces in the total amount of water, then turn off the heat and add the light pieces to the same pot. Let steep for another five to thirty minutes (usually fifteen), the time depending on the strength your taste buds will tolerate, and strain. The usual range of tea dose is ½ to 1 cup of tea two or three times a day. You can increase the dosage for stronger short-term effects (two to seven days).

Congratulations—you have blended your own herbal tea! The effort you have put into creating it will repay you a hundredfold in natural healing consistent with your own special needs.

Herbal Home Medicine Chest

Most minor health problems can be handled with a few dried herbs for teas, a few concentrates, or the compounds, such as herb salves. The twenty-one herbs in the list that follows provide tried-and-true relief for simple maladies. Each can be used for a few different things. All are readily available, are safe when used as described in this book, and are excellent candidates for a home medicine chest.

By all means, customize your medicine chest as needed—for example, you may want to substitute herbs that grow abundantly in your vicinity or that are effective for the most common problems that recur in your household. The important thing is to not get too many herbs in the house at once so you can learn about the ones you have and more readily maintain a fresh supply. Once you get to know the herbs in your home medicine chest, you'll find that they're as terrific as they sound.

Note that glycerin-based tinctures are occasionally recommended in the list to avoid alcohol, to provide a more pleasant taste, or to improve the herb's beneficial effect; however, it really doesn't matter whether you prefer to use tinctures, glycerin-based tinctures, capsules, or tablets. Follow dosages given on product labels or recommendations in the pages where these herbs are mentioned earlier in this book.

HERB	ACTIONS	USES
Chaste berry seed, tincture	Emmenagogue Hormonal normalizer	For late period For irregular cycle
Comfrey root and leaf, dried, for external compresses and poultices	Vulnerary	For superficial wounds or deep bruises
Cramp bark, tincture	Antispasmodic	For cramps
Dandelion leaf and root, for tea; or fresh leaves in spring, juiced	Diuretic	For water retention
Eleutherococcus (formerly known as Siberian ginseng), tincture	Adaptogen	For energy, endurance, or coping with stress
Fennel, dried seed, for tea	Carminative	For gas
Garlic, as food or in deodorized capsules	Antimicrobial	For poor immune response
Hawthorn flower, leaf, and berry, for tea or tincture; also berry jam	Heart tonic	For weakness of the heart

HERB	ACTIONS	USES
Lavender, essential oil, externally	Antidepressant aromatherapy	For immediate relief
	Antiseptic	For a wound or an infection of the skin
Marshmallow, dried root, for tea or syrup	Demulcent	For irritation with symptoms, inside or out
Nettle, dried, for tea and syrup	Tonic	If you seem to need everything all at once
Peppermint, dried, for tea	Antacid	Instead of bicarbonates
Raspberry leaf, dried, for tea	Uterine tonic	For pregnancy or a need to heal the womb
Sarsaparilla, tea or tincture	Alterative	For chronic hormonal, lymph, or skin problems
Skullcap, tincture	Nervine relaxant	For tension headache
St. John's wort, tincture	Antidepressant	If you have eight weeks or more to uplift mood
Valerian, glycerin tincture	Analgesic	For pain
	Hypnotic	For insomnia
Wild oats, tincture from fresh plant in "milky" stage	Nervine tonic	For nervous exhaustion
Wild yam, glycerin tincture	Anti-inflammatory	For inflammation
Yarrow, dried flower, for tea	Astringent	For diarrhea, discharge, or blood loss
	Bitter	For poor digestion
Yellow dock, dried root, for tea; or glycerin tincture	Aperient, laxative	For constipation

appendix d
Herb Images

Herbal medicine is more than chemical constituents and research studies. From the beginning of time, scholars of medicinal plant use have meditated on the morphology, or form, of our remedies. Sitting with and growing live plants repays time spent with plant knowledge that will never be reduced to words written in books or spoken. Pictures are another way to bring plants, with their often-strange names, into our nonverbal experience. These illustrations represent many of the herbs in formulas contained in this book.

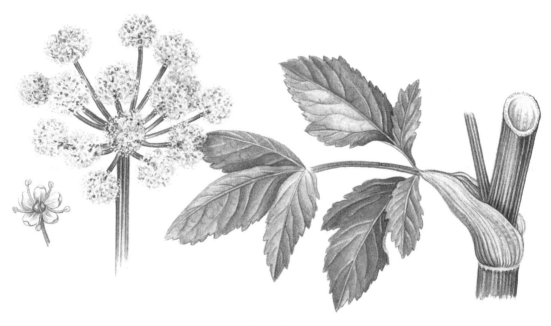

Angelica

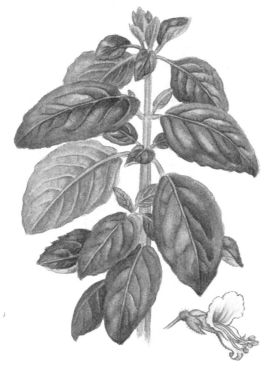

Basil

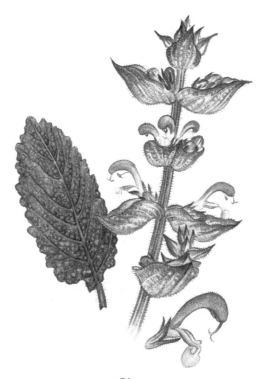

Clary

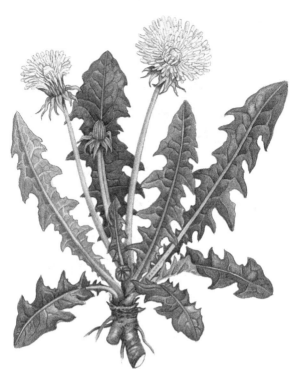

Dandelion

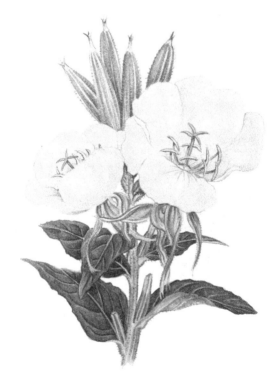

Evening Primrose

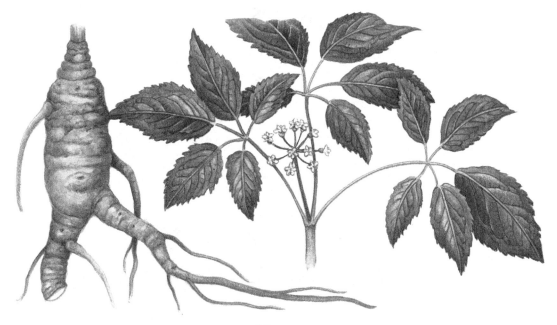

Ginseng

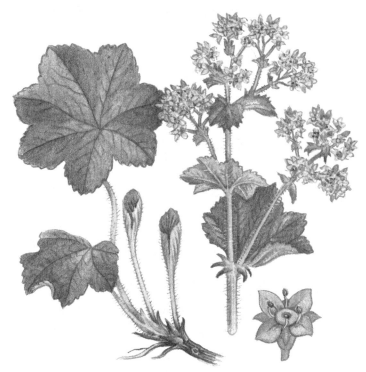

Lady's Mantle

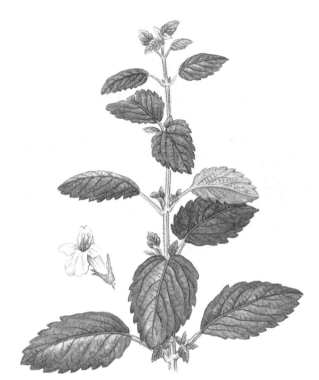

Lemon Balm

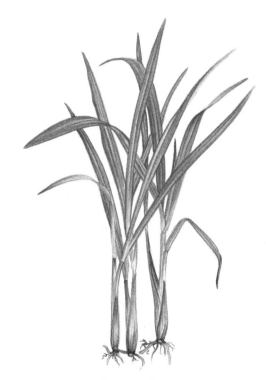

Lemon Grass

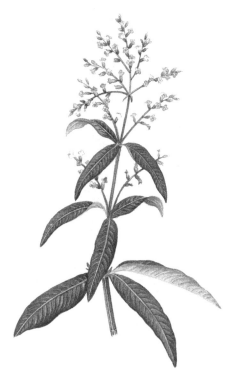

Lemon Verbena

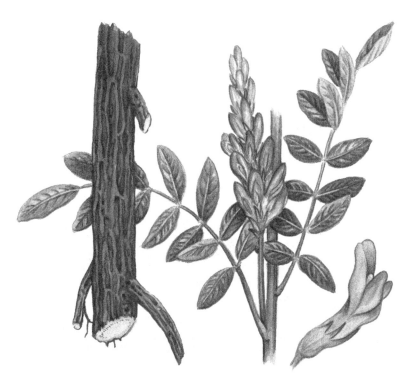

Licorice

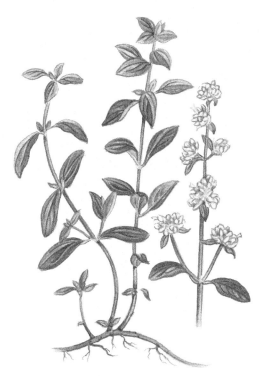

Marjoram

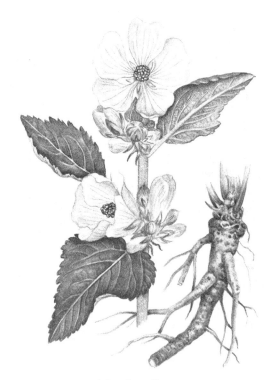

Marshmallow

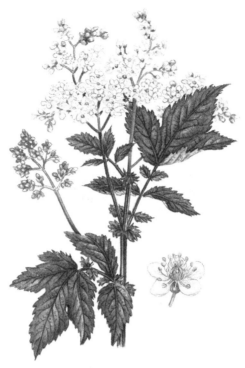

Meadowsweet

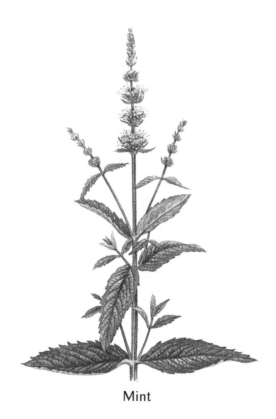

Mint

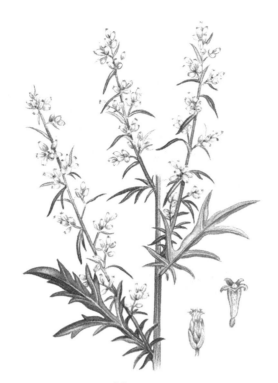

Mugwort

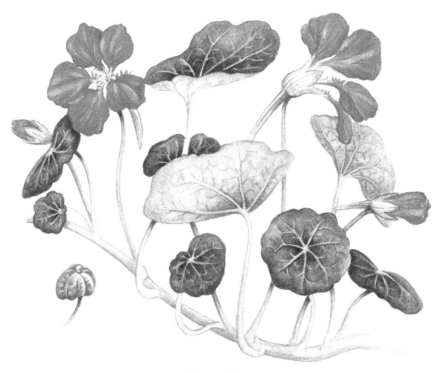

Nasturtium

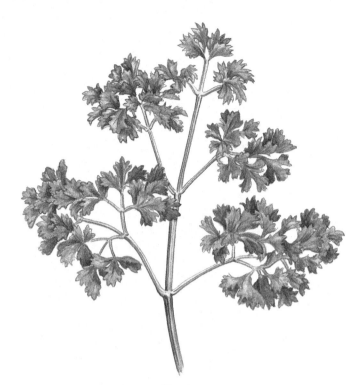

Parsley

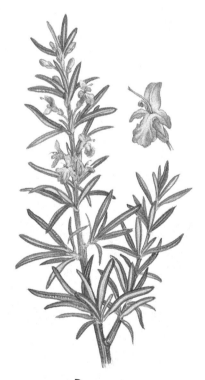

Rosemary

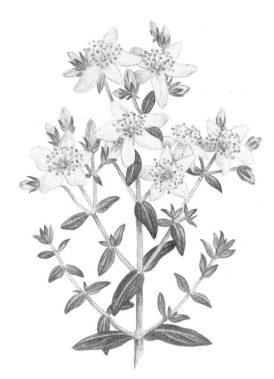

St. John's Wort

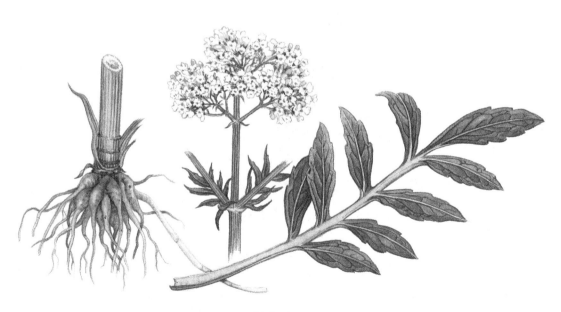

Valerian

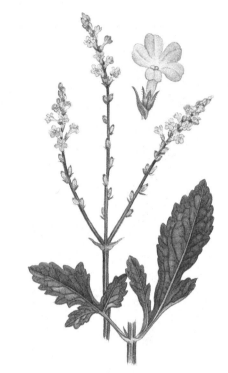

Vervain

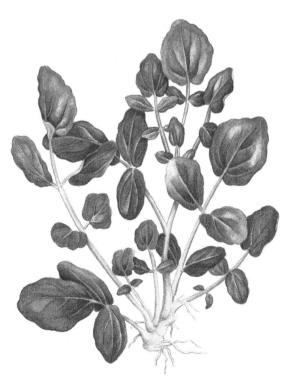

Watercress

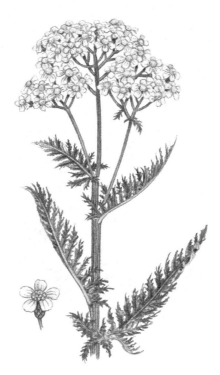

Yarrow

Resources

More than any other part of this book, the resources for herbal medicine continue to change. For those readers who are online, the simplest gateway to all things herbal is www.herbnet.com, the first listed resource here. For others who prefer to contact companies without the use of a computer, I have listed a few resources. Herbalists often teach classes and offer a wide variety of health services. Professional organizations, including those listed below, can give referrals to herbalists, naturopaths, acupuncturists, midwives, and other natural health-care providers in your area.

THE HERB GROWING & MARKETING NETWORK

Maureen Rogers, Director
PO Box 245
Silver Spring, MD 17575
(717) 393-3295
www.herbnet.com

The Herbal Green Pages
This "green phone book" is the most complete resource for herbs, herbalists, teachers, herb products, everything in the world to do with herbs, and herb-related links and publications.

Companies from All Regions

ADAPTATIONS

Tane & Maureen Datta
PO Box 1070
Captain Cook, HI 96704
(808) 324-6600

Tropical, high-quality organic herbs, foods, available wholesale and retail; customer pays for shipping from Hawaii.

AVENA BOTANICALS

Deb Soule
219 Mill Street
Rockport, ME 04856
(207) 594-0694
www.avenabotanicals.com

Teaching, gifted herb grower, formulator, woman-owned and woman-operated herbal apothecary offering organic teas and a wide assortment of products.

BISBEE BOTANICALS

PO Box 218
Gila, NM 88038
(505) 535-4352

Single herb extracts, oils; specializes in ecologically gathered southwestern plants.

BLESSED BOTANICALS

Tara Lee Fitzgibbon
770 Briar Ridge Road
Burnsville, NC 28714
(828) 682-7226

www.blessedbotanicals.com
An array of herb tea blends to delight any palate.

BLESSED HERBS, INC.

109 Barre Plains Road
Oakham, MA 01068
(800) 489-4372
(508) 882-3839

Huge range of common and uncommon herb products.

EARTH'S HARVEST, INC.

14385 S.E. Lusted Road
Sandy, OR 97055
(800) 952-7921
(503) 668-4120
www.aminoacidbotanicalandsupplementsource.net/
EarthsHarvest.htm

Herbal salves and more.

FOSTER'S BOTANICAL AND HERB REVIEWS

PO Box 191
Eureka Springs, AR 72632
(479) 253-2629
www.stevenfoster.com

Consulting, photography, and publications, specializing in medicinal and aromatic plants.

GAIA HERBS

101 Gaia Herbs Drive
Brevard, NC 28712
(800) 831-7780
www.gaiaherbs.com

A large herb company providing excellent products, retail and wholesale, with links to conferences.

HERBALIST & ALCHEMIST

David Winston
(908) 689-9020
www.herbalist-alchemist.com

Traditional Chinese, Native American, Western herbs, classes, and rare herb books.

HERBPHARM

Ed Smith
PO Box 116
Williams, OR 97544
(541) 846-6262

Retail and professional line of organic, wild-crafted extracts, combinations, oils from around the world; also internships and books.

HERBS ETC.

Daniel Gagnon
1345 Cerrillos Road
Santa Fe, NM 87505
(888) 694-3727
www.herbsetc.com

One of the best herbal supplement companies widely available in retail outlets and by mail order; wide variety of products.

ISLAND HERBS

Ryan Drum
PO Box 25
Waldron Island, WA 98297-0025
www.ryandrum.com

Teaching, and the best dried red clover, nettles, kelp, edible seaweeds; many other organic, dried medicinal herbs.

MOONMAID BOTANICALS

Cynthia Johnston
Cosby, TN 37722
(877) 253-7853
www.moonmaidbotanicals.com

Delicious face creams and more.

MOUNTAIN ROSE HERBS

PO Box 50220
Eugene, OR 97405
(800) 879-3337
www.mountainroseherbs.com

Wide selection of bulk herbs and supplies.

OAK VALLEY HERB FARM

Kathi Keville
14648 Pear Tree Lane
Nevada City, CA 95959
(916) 265-9552
www.ahaherb.com

Editor of the best all-around herb newsletter, the *American Herb Association Quarterly*. Classes; excellent-quality dried herbs and essential oils; books.

PROFESSIONAL COMPLEMENTARY HEALTH FORMULAS, INC.

Hugh and Martha Helikson
PO Box 80085
Portland, OR 92780
(800) 952-2219
www.professionalformulas.com

The supplier of Amanda's herbal menopause formula, Graceful Change, in capsules, plus single herbs, homeopathic medicine, and nutritional supplements.

RED MOON HERBS

Corinna Woods
(888) 929-0777
www.redmoonherbs.com

High-quality salves and other products, links to conferences, teaching.

UNITEA HERBS

PO Box 8005, Suite 318
Boulder, CO 80306
(303) 443-1248

Delicious tea blends for pleasure and for hard-bitten coffee fans and herb skeptics.

VITALITY WORKS

8409 Washington Street NE
Albuquerque, NM 87113
(505) 268-9950
www.vitalityworks.com

Herbal formulas, extracts, and oils.

WOODLAND ESSENCE

Kate Gilday
392 Teacup Street
Cold Brook, NY 13324
(315) 845-1515
www.woodlandessence.com

Teaching and products, especially the herbal balm called Love Butter.

Other Herb Centers, Organizations, and Further Studies

AMERICAN BOTANICAL COUNCIL

PO Box 201660
Austin, TX 78720
(512) 331-1924
www.herbalgram.org

Publishes *HerbGram* magazine, textbooks on herbal medicine, and scientific herb studies.

AMERICAN HERB ASSOCIATION

Kathi Keville
PO Box 16733
Nevada City, CA 95959
(530) 265-9552
www.ahaherb.com

Membership offers many benefits, including the best practical, low-cost clinical herbalism newsletter, *American Herb Association Quarterly Newsletter*. Teaching, how-to articles, herb products, exquisite essential oils from her company, Oak Valley Herb Farm.

AMERICAN HERBAL PHARMACOPOEIA

Roy Upton, Editor
PO Box 66809
Scotts Valley, CA 95067
(831) 461-6318
www.herbal-ahp.org

Peer-reviewed herb monographs, pharmacognosy and clinical data, analytical testing.

AMERICAN HERBALISTS GUILD

141 Nob Hill Road
Cheshire, CT 06410
(203) 272-6731
www.americanherbalist.com

The guild's directory of herbal education programs is the most complete listing of educational programs available to date. Categorized by state; includes residential and correspondence programs; specifies programs' focus (such as Western). Also lists publications, computer networks, and events. The membership directory provides referrals to practicing professional herbalists.

AMERICAN HOLISTIC HEALTH ASSOCIATION

PO Box 17400
Anaheim, CA 92817
(714) 779-6152
www.ahha.org

Call for information and referrals.

BLAZING STAR HERBAL SCHOOL

Tony(a) Lemos, Director
PO Box 6
Shelburne Falls, MA 01370
(413) 625-6875
www.blazingstarherbalschool.org

Teaching, books, children's herbs, politically aware environmental herbal medicine, international food activism, and peace work/play.

THE EUROPEAN HERBAL AND TRADITIONAL MEDICINE PRACTITIONERS ALLIANCE

EHTPA
25 Lincoln Close
Tewkesbury
Glos
Gloucestershire, UK
GL20 5TY
info@ehpa.eu

Represents professional organizations of herbal practitioners throughout Europe.

HERB RESEARCH FOUNDATION

4140 15th Street
Boulder, CO 80304
(303) 449-2265
www.herbs.org

Literature searches, more than 300,000 articles, answers to herb questions from a scientific perspective.

NATIONAL HERBALISTS ASSOCIATION OF AUSTRALIA

PO Box 45
Concord West
NSW
2138
Australia
(02) 8765-0071
www.nhaa.org.au

Professional organization of herbalists offers referrals in Australia, conferences. Publishes *Australian Journal of Medical Herbalism*.

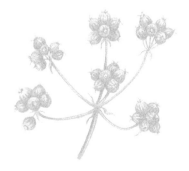

THE NATIONAL INSTITUTE OF MEDICAL HERBALISTS

Elm House
54 Mary Arches Street
Exeter
EX4 3BA
UK
+44 (0) 1392 426022
info@nimh.org.uk

Britain's professional herbalists' organization; offers information on training, referrals throughout the world.

NORTHEAST HERBAL ASSOCIATION

PO Box 294
Ashville, MA 01330
neha@northeastherbal.org

The association's membership directory provides referrals to wonderful herbalists, teachers, resources, and companies offering herb products.

ONTARIO HERBALISTS ASSOCIATION

PO Box 123
Station D
Etobicoke, Ontario
M9A 4X2
Canada
1-877-OHA-HERB (1-877-642-4372)
(416) 236-0090
info@herbalists.on.ca

Referrals to professional members, businesses. Publishes *Canadian Journal of Herbalism*.

PARTNER EARTH EDUCATION CENTER

Pam Montgomery
Sweetwater Sanctuary
1525 Danby Mountain Road
Danby, VT 05739
(802) 293-5996
www.partnereartheducationcenter.com

Teaching, healing, envisioning. Author of the bestselling book *Plant Spirit Healing*.

SAGE

Rosemary Gladstar
PO Box 420
East Barre, VT 05649
(802) 479-9825
www.sagemountain.com

Teaching, products, conferences, and international herbal travel adventures.

THE SELF-HEAL SCHOOL OF HERBAL STUDIES AND HEALING

John Finch and Jane Richmond
PO Box 70131
San Diego, CA 92167
(619) 224-1268
www.selfhealschool.com

Teaching, conferences, healings, herbal consultations, herb walks, and the world's best herbal sports balm, plus fantastic beauty cream.

UNITED PLANT SAVERS

PO Box 400
East Barre, VT 05649
(802) 476-6467
info@unitedplantsavers.org

A nonprofit organization for replanting and protecting endangered plants, including medicinal herbs threatened by development. Herbalists rely on their updates to change our use of herbs for the sake of biodiversity.

WISE WOMAN CENTER

Susun Weed
PO Box 64
Woodstock, NY 12498
(845) 246-8081
www.susunweed.com

Teaching, empowerment of the wisdom in each woman, books, apprenticeships, and more than can be told here.

Herbal Education on Television or Audio/Videotape

CREATIVE SEMINARS
PO Box 203
West Hurley, NY 12491
(845) 679-6885
www.cstapes.com

Taped seminars on herbs, nutrition, and natural health; includes many of Amanda's past and recent lectures.

THE NATIONAL INSTITUTES OF HEALTH
Office of Alternative Medicine
6120 Executive Plaza South, Room 450
Rockville, MD 20092
(301) 402-2466

Information on research into traditional medicines using plants and other natural therapies.

NORTH AMERICAN INSTITUTE OF MEDICAL HERBALISM
2900 Valmont Road
Boulder, CO 80301
(720) 406-8609
naimh.org
medherb.com

Teaching, compelling Web resources; *Medical Herbalism* newsletter.

THE SOUTHWEST SCHOOL OF BOTANIC MEDICINE
Founded by Michael Moore
Donna Chesner, Administrator
www.swsbm.com

The premier Web source for herb manuals, teaching, plant photographs, historical botanic medicine writings, and the genius of the late Michael Roland Shaw Moore.

TREE FARM COMMUNICATIONS
23703 NE 4th Street
Sammamish, WA 98074
(800) 468-0464
(425) 868-0464
info@treefarmtapes.com

Video and audiotapes of all aspects of health; includes many of Amanda's past and recent lectures.

WHAT A RELIEF!
HOSTED BY AMANDA MCQUADE CRAWFORD
www.veria.com

Distributed by DISH and Verizon FIOS.

Websites

INTERNATIONAL MENOPAUSE SOCIETY
www.imsociety.org

LONGWOOD HERBAL TASK FORCE
www.mcp.edu/herbal

NATIONAL OSTEOPOROSIS SOCIETY
www.nos.org.uk

NATIONAL WOMEN'S HEALTH INFORMATION CENTER
www.4woman.gov

Website of the Office of Women's Health in the United States Department of Health and Human Services.

NATIONAL WOMEN'S HEALTH NETWORK
www.womenshealthnetwork.org

The best single site for newest and balanced health updates on menopause.

NORTH AMERICA MENOPAUSE SOCIETY
www.menopause.org

Bibliography

Abenhaim, H., and B. L. Harlow. "*The Harvard Study of Moods and Cycles.*" *Archives of General Psychiatry* 63 (2006): 385–90.

Abraham, G. E. "Nutritional Factors in the Etiology of PMS." *Journal of Reproductive Medicine* 28, no. 7 (1983): 446–64.

Adami, S., L. Bufalino, R. Cervetti. "Ipriflavone Prevents Radial Bone Loss in Postmenopausal Women with Low Bone Mass over 2 Years." *Osteoporosis International* 7 (1997): 119.

Agnusdei, D., G. Crepaldi, G. Isaia. "A Double-Blind Placebo-Controlled Trial of Ipriflavone for Prevention of Postmenopausal Spinal Bone Loss." *Calcified Tissue International* 61, Suppl. (1997): 19.

Akhondzadeh, S., H. R. Naghavi, M. Vazirian, et al. "Passionflower in the Treatment of Generalized Anxiety: A Pilot Double-Blind Randomized Controlled Trial with Oxazepam." *Journal of Clinical Pharmacy and Therapeutics* 26, no. 5 (2001): 363.

Albertazzi, P., F. Pansini, G. Bonaccorsi, et al. "The Effect of Dietary Soy Supplementation on Hot Flashes." *Obstetrics and Gynecology* 91 (1998): 6–11.

Ally, M. M. "The Pharmacological Action of *Zingiber officinale*," in *Proceedings of the 4th Pan Indian Ocean Scientific Congress,* Karachi, Pakistan, Section G, 11–12, 1960.

Asimov, I. *The Human Body.* New York: Mentor, 1963.

Barnes, S., and T. G. Peterson. "Biochemical Targets of the Isoflavone Genistein in Tumor Cell Lines." *Proceedings of the Society for Experimental Biology and Medicine* 208, no. 1 (1995): 10–38.

Barnhart, E., pub. *Physician's Desk Reference.* Oradell, NJ: Medical Economics Data, 1992.

Becker, P. "Insomnia: Prevalence, Impact, Pathogenesis, Differential Diagnosis, and Evaluation." *Psychiatric Clinics of North America* 29 (2006): 855–870.

Beckham, N. "Phyto-oestrogens and Compounds That Affect Oestrogen Metabolism." *Australian Journal of Medical Herbalism* 7, no. 1 (1995): 11–16; no. 2 (1995): 27–33.

Bergner, P., ed. "Chaste-Tree *(Vitex aganus-castus)*." *Medical Herbalism* 2, no. 5 (1990): 1, 6.

Berkow, R., et al. *Merck Manual,* 15th ed. Rahway, NJ: Merck & Co., 1987.

Bianchi, G., et al. "Effects of Gonadotrophin-releasing Hormone Agonist on Uterine Fibroids and Bone Density." *Maturitas* 11 (1989): 179–85.

Blumenthal, M. *The ABC Clinical Guide to Herbs.* New York: Thieme Press, 2002.

Blumenthal, M. "Systematic Reviews and Meta-Analyses Support the Efficacy of Numerous Popular Herbs and Phytomedicines." *Alternative Therapies in Health and Medicine* 15, no. 2 (2009): 14–15.

Bonaiuti, D., B. Shea, R. Iovine, S. Negrini. "Exercise for Preventing and Treating Osteoporosis in Postmenopausal Women." *Cochrane Reviews,* The Cochrane Library, 2003.

Borer, K. "Physical Activity in the Prevention and Amelioration of Osteoporosis in Women: Interaction of Mechanical, Hormonal and Dietary Factors." *Sports Medicine* 35, no. 9 (2005): 779–830.

Brown, M. A., and J. Robinson. *When Your Body Gets the Blues: The Clinically Proven Program for Women Who Feel Tired and Stressed and Eat Too Much.* New York: Berkley, 2002.

Burdette, J. E., J. Liu, S. N. Chen, et al. "Black Cohosh Acts as a Mixed Competitive Ligand and Partial Agonist of the Serotonin Receptor." *Journal of Agricultural and Food Chemistry* 51, no. 19 (2003): 5661–5670.

Butterweck, V. "Mechanism of Action of St. John's Wort in Depression: What Is Known?" *CNS Drugs* 17, no. 8 (2003): 539–562.

Carey, C. "Disorders of Sexual Desire and Arousal." *Obstetrics and Gynecology Clinics of North America* 33 (2006): 549–564.

Carroll, D. G. "Nonhormonal Therapies for Hot Flashes in Menopause." *American Family Physician* 73, no. 3 (2006): 457–464.

Cashman, K. "Diet, Nutrition, and Bone Health." *Experimental Biology and Medicine (Maywood)* 232 (2007): 1275–1288.

Cassidy, A., P. Albertazzi, and I. Nielsen. "Critical Review of Health Effects of Soybean Phyto-oestrogens in Postmenopausal Women." *Proceedings of the Nutrition Society* 65 (2006): 76–92.

Center, C., M. Davis, T. Detre, et al. "Confronting Depression and Suicide in Physicians: A Consensus Statement." *Journal of the American Medical Association* 289, no. 23 (2003): 3161–66.

Colbin, A. *Food and Healing.* New York: Ballantine, 1986.

"Consensus Statement on Progestin Use in Postmenopausal Women." Editorial. *Maturitas* 11 (1988): 175–77.

Coombs, N. J., et al. *"HRT and Breast Cancer: Impact on Population Risk and Incidence." European Journal of Cancer* 41, no. 12 (2005): 1775–81.

Cranney, A., H. Weiler, S. O'Donnell, and L. Puil. "Summary of Evidence-Based Review on Vitamin D Efficacy and Safety in Relation to Bone Health." *The American Journal of Clinical Nutrition* 88, Suppl. (2008): 513S–9S.

Culbreth, D. *Manual of Materia Medica and Pharmacology.* Sandy, OR: Eclectic Institute, 1927.

Cuzick, J. *"Hormone Replacement Therapy and the Risk of Breast Cancer." European Journal of Cancer* 44, no. 16 (2008): 2344–49.

Das, S., et al. *"Long-Term Effects of Energy-Restricted Diets Differing in Glycemic Load on Metabolic Adaptation and Body Composition." Open Nutrition Journal* 2 (2008): 76–85.

Dennerstein, L., P. Lehert, E. Dudley, et al. "Factors Contributing to Positive Mood during the Menopausal Transition." *The Journal of Nervous and Mental Disease* 189, no. 2 (2001): 84–89.

Dentali, S. "Hormones and Yams." *American Herb Association Quarterly Newsletter* 10, no. 4 (1994).

Dhawan, K., S. Dhawan, A. Sharma. "Passiflora: A Review Update." *Journal of Ethnopharmacology* 94, no. 1 (2004): 1–23.

Ding, E., S. Hutfless, X. Ding, and S. Girota. "Chocolate and the Prevention of Cardiovascular Disease." *Nutrition & Metabolism* 2, no. 2 (2006): 1–12.

Ellingwood, R. *American Materia Medica, Therapeutics and Pharmacognosy.* Portland, OR: Eclectic Medical Pubs., 1983.

Engelsen, J., J. D. Nielsen, K. F. Hansen. "Effect of Coenzyme Q10 and Ginkgo Biloba on Warfarin Dosage in Patients on Long-Term Warfarin Treatment: A Randomized, Double-Blind Placebo-Controlled Crossover Trial." *Ugeskr Laeger* 165, no. 18 (2003): 1868–71.

Erdman, J. W. Jr., T. M. Badger, J. W. Lampe, et al. "Not All Soy Products Are Created Equal: Caution Needed in Interpretation of Research Results." *Journal of Nutrition* 134, no. 5 (2004): 1229S–33S.

Evans, F. J., ed. *British Herbal Pharmacopoeia.* Bournemouth, UK: Megaron Press, 1983.

Felter, H. W. *The Eclectic Materia Medica, Pharmacology and Therapeutics,* reprint, 1922. Portland, OR: Eclectic Medical Pubs., 1983.

Felter, H. W., and J. U. Lloyd. *King's American Dispensatory,* 18th ed., 2 vols. 1898. Sandy, OR: Eclectic Medical Pubs., 1983.

Feng, J., and G. MacGregor. "Beneficial Effects of Potassium on Human Health." *Physiologia Plantarum* 133 (2008): 725–735.

Fletcher, S. W., and G. Colditz. "Failure of Oestrogen Plus Progestin Therapy for Prevention." *Journal of the American Medical Association* 288 (2002): 366–368.

Foster, S., and J. Duke. *Eastern/Central Medicinal Plants.* Peterson Field Guide Series. Boston: Houghton Mifflin, 1990.

Freudenstein, J., C. Dasenbrock, T. Nisslein. "Lack of Promotion of Estrogen-Dependent Mammary Gland Tumors in Vivo by an Isopropanolic *Cimicifuga racemosa* Extract." *Cancer Research* 62, no. 12 (2002): 3448–52.

Fugh-Berman, A. "Black Cohosh." *The Five-Minute Herb & Dietary Supplement Consult.* Philadelphia: Lippincott, Williams & Wilkins, 2003.

Gaby, A. "Multi-level Yam Scam." *American Herb Association Quarterly Newsletter* 12, no. 1 (1996).

Garland, S. *The Herb Garden.* New York: Penguin, 1984.

Geller, S. E., and L. Studee. "Botanical and Dietary Supplements for Menopausal Symptoms: What Works, What Does Not." *Journal of Women's Health* 14, no. 7 (2005): 634–49.

Greenspan, M. *Healing Through the Dark Emotions: The Wisdom of Grief, Fear, and Despair.* Boston: Shambhala, 2003.

Grieves, M. *Modern Herbal.* New York: Dover, 1933.

Gunn, J. D. *New Domestic Physician or, Home Book of Health.* Cincinnati: Moore, Wilstach, & Keys, 1861.

Guttuso, T., R. Kurlan, M. McDermott, et al. "Gabapentin's Effects on Hot Flashes in Postmenopausal Women: A Randomized Controlled Trial." *Obstetrics and Gynecology* 101 (2003): 337.

Hadley, S., and J. J. Petry. "Valerian." *American Family Physician* 67, no. 8 (2003): 1155–58.

Hahn, G., et al. "Monchspfeffer (Monkspepper)." *Notabene Medici* 16 (1986): 233–6, 297–301.

Hammerness, P., E. Basch, C. Ulbricht, et al. "St. John'sWwort: A Systematic Review of Adverse Effects and Drug Interactions for the Consultation Psychiatrist." *Psychosomatics* 44, no. 4 (2003): 271–82.

Hernandez, Munoz, G., and S. Pluchino. "*Cimicifuga racemosa* for the Treatment of Hot Flashes in Women Surviving Breast Cancer." *Maturitas* 44, Suppl 1 (2003): S59–65.

Herrington, D., and T. Howard. "From Presumed Benefit to Potential Harm[—]Hormone Therapy and Heart Disease." *New England Journal of Medicine.* 349, no. 6 (2003): 519–21.

Hidalgo, L. A., P. A. Chedraui, N. Morocho, et al. "The Effect of Red Clover Isoflavones on Menopausal Symptoms, Lipids, and Vaginal Cytology in Menopausal Women: A Randomized, Double-Blind Placebo-Controlled Study." *Gynecological Endocrinology* 21, no. 5 (2005): 257–64.

Hobbs, C. "Vitex: The Female Herb." *The American Herb Association Quarterly Newsletter* VII, no. 3 (1990): 5.

Hoerhammer, L., et al. "Chemistry, Pharmacology, and Pharmaceutics of the Components from *Viburnum prunifolium and V. opulus.*" *Botanical Magazine* (Tokyo) 79 (1966): 510–25.

Hoffmann, D. *Medical Herbalism: The Science and Practice of Herbal Medicine.* Rochester, VT: Healing Arts Press, 2003.

Horrobin, D. F. "The Role of Essential Fatty Acids and Prostaglandins in the Premenstrual Syndrome." *Journal of Reproductive Medicine* 28, no. 7 (1983): 465–68.

Houck, J. A. *Hot and Bothered: Women, Medicine and Menopause in Modern America.* Cambridge: Harvard University Press, 2006.

Hu, Z., X. Yang, P. C. L. Ho, et al. "Herb-Drug Interactions: A Literature review." *Drugs* 65, no. 9 (2005): 1239–82.

Huntley, A., and E. Ernst. "A Systematic Review of the Safety of Black Cohosh." *Menopause* 10, no. 1 (2003): 58–64.

Jarboe, C. H., et al. "Uterine Relaxant Properties of Viburnum." *Nature* 212, no. 5064 (1966): 837.

Jarry, H., M. Metten, B. Spengler, et al. "In Vitro Effects of the *Cimicifuga racemosa* extract BNO 1055." *Maturitas* 44, Suppl 1 (2003): S31–38.

Jenkins, V., et. al. "*Does Endocrine Therapy for the Treatment and Prevention of Breast Cancer Affect Memory and Cognition?*" *European Journal of Cancer* 43, no. 9 (2007): 1342–47.

Kalus, J. S., A. A. Piotrowski, C. R. Fortier, et al. "Hemodynamic and Electrocardiographic Effects of Short-Term Ginkgo Biloba." *Annals of Pharmacotherapy* 37, no. 3 (2003): 345–49.

Kaptchuk, T. *The Web That Has No Weaver.* New York: Congdon & Weed, 1983.

Kennedy, D., W. Little, and A. Scholey. "Effects of *Melissa officinalis* (Lemon Balm) on Mood Changes during Acute Psychological Stress." *Pharmacology, Biochemistry, and Behavior* 72 (2003): 953–64.

Keville, K. *Illustrated Herb Encyclopedia.* New York: Mallard, 1991.

———, ed. "GLA Studies." *American Herb Association Quarterly Newsletter* 4, no. 4 (1986): 16.

Kligler, B. "Black Cohosh." *American Family Physician* 68, no. 1 (2003): 114–16.

Krebs, E. E., K. E. Ensrud, R. MacDonald, et al. "Phytoestrogens for Treatment of Menopausal Symptoms: A Systematic Review." *Obstetrics and Gynecology* 104, no. 4 (2004): 824–36.

Kubota, S., and S. Nakashima. "The Study of *Leonurus sibericus L. ii.* Pharmacological Study of the Alkaloid 'Leonurin' Isolated from *Leonurus sibericus L.*" *Folia Pharmacologica Japonica* 11, no. 2 (1930): 159–67.

Kuroda, K., and T. Kaku. "Pharmacological and Chemical Studies on the Alcohol Extract of *Capsella bursa-pastoris.*" *Life Sciences* 8, no. 3 (1969): 151–55.

Kuroda, K., and K. Takagi. "Physiologically Active Substances in *Capsella bursa-pastoris*." *Nature* 220, no. 5168 (1968): 707–8.

Lee, J. R. "Osteoporosis Reversal: The Role of Progesterone." *International Clinical Nutrition Review* 10, no. 3 (1990): 384–91.

———, and V. Hopkins. *What Your Doctor May Not Tell You about Menopause.*New York: Warner Books, 2004.

Levitsky, J., T. A. Alli, J. Wisecarver, et al. "Fulminant Liver Failure Associated with the Use of Black Cohosh." *Digestive Diseases and Sciences* 50, no. 3 (2005): 538–39.

Li, C., K. Malone, P. Porter, et al. "Relationship between Long Durations and Different Regimens of Hormone Therapy and Risk of Breast Cancer." *Journal of the American Medical Association* 289, no. 24 (2003): 3254–63.

Love, S. *Dr. Susan Love's Hormone Book.* New York: Random House, 1997.

Lupattelli, G., S. Marchesi, R. Lombardini, et al. "Artichoke Juice Improves Endothelial Function in Hyperlipemia." *Life Sciences* 76, no. 7 (2004): 775–82.

Lutomski, J. "Chemistry and the Therapeutic Use of Licorice *(Glycyrrhiza glabra L.)*." *Pharmazie in Unserer Zeit* 12, no. 2 (1983): 49–54.

Mabey, R., ed. *The New Age Herbalist.* New York: Macmillan, Collier, 1988.

Mahady, G.B. "Black Cohosh *(Actaea/Cimicifuga racemosa)*: Review of the Clinical Data for Safety and Efficacy in Menopausal Symptoms." *Treatments in Endocrinology* 4, no. 3 (2005): 177–84.

Manson, J., J. Hsia, K. Johnson, et al. "Estrogen Plus Progestin and the Risk of Coronary Heart Disease." *New England Journal of Medicine* 349, no. 6 (2003): 523–34.

McIntyre, A. *Herbs for Common Ailments.* New York: Simon & Schuster, Element Books, 1992.

McQuade, Crawford, A. "Menopause—Graceful Rite of Change." *Essays on Herbalism,* vol. 2. Edited by Michael Tierra. Englewood Cliffs, NJ: Prentice Hall, in press.

———. "The Role of Phytosterols in Women's Health." Symposium lecture, Breitenbush Herb Retreat, Breitenbush, OR, 1989.

Meisenbach Boylan, K. *The Seven Sacred Rites of Menopause: The Spiritual Journey to the Wise-Woman Years.* Santa Monica: Santa Monica Press, 2000.

Mellman, T. "Sleep and Anxiety Disorders." *Psychiatric Clinics of North America* 29 (2006): 1047–58.

Mills, S. *The Dictionary of Modern Herbalism: A Comprehensive Guide to Practical Herbal Therapy.* Rochester, VT: Healing Arts Press, 1988.

———, and K. Bone. *The Essential Guide to Herbal Safety.* St. Louis: Churchill Livingstone, 2005.

Minciullo, P. L., A. Saija, M. Patafi, et al. "Muscle Damage Induced by Black Cohosh *(Cimicifuga racemosa)*." *Phytomedicine* 13, no. 1–2 (2006): 115–18.

Moore, M. *Medicinal Plants of the Desert and Canyon West.* Santa Fe: Museum of New Mexico Press, 1989.

———. *Medicinal Plants of the Mountain West.* Santa Fe: Museum of New Mexico Press, 1979.

———. *Medicinal Plants of the Pacific West.* Santa Fe: Red Crane Books, 1993.

Moore, M., and D. Gagnon. *Clinical Herbal Repertory.* Self-published, 1986.

Moss, M., J. Cook, K. Wesnes, and P. Duckett. "Aromas of Rosemary and Lavender Essential Oils Differentially Affect Cognition and Mood in Healthy Adults." *International Journal of Neuroscience* 113, no. 1 (2003): 15–38.

Mowrey, D. *The Scientific Validation of Herbal Medicine.* N.p.: Cormorant Books, 1986.

Moynihan, R. "The Marketing of a Disease: Female Sexual Dysfunction." *British Medical Journal* 330, no. 7484 (2005): 192–94.

Murray, M., and J. Pizzorno. *Encyclopedia of Natural Medicine.* Rocklin, CA: Prima, 1990.

Nelson, H. D., K. K. Vesco, E. Haney, et al. "Nonhormonal Therapies for Menopausal Hot Flashes: Systematic Review and Meta-Analysis." *Journal of the American Medical Association* 295, no. 17 (2006): 2057–71.

Northrup, C. *The Wisdom of Menopause.* New York: Bantam Books, 2001.

Northrup, C. *Women's Bodies, Women's Wisdom.* New York: Bantam Books, 1994.

Notelovitz, M., and M. Ware. *Stand Tall! Preventing Osteoporosis.* Gainesville, FL: Triad, 1982.

Ottem, D. P., L. K. Carr, A. E. Perks, P. Lee, and J. M. H. Teichman. "Interstitial Cystitis and Female Sexual Dysfunction." *Urology* 69 (2007): 4608–10.

Paul, M. *The Women's Pharmacy.* New York: Simon & Schuster, Cornerstone Library, 1983.

Pearson, C., et al. *Taking Hormones and Women's Health—Choices, Risks and Benefits.* Washington, DC: National Women's Health Network, 1995.

Percy, E. C., and J. D. Carson. "The Use of DMSO in Tennis Elbow and Rotator Cuff Tendinitis: A Double-Blind Study." *Medicine and Science in Sports and Exercise* 13 (1981): 215–19.

Perez, D. G., and C. L Loprinzi. "Newer Antidepressants and Other Nonhormonal Agents for the Treatment of Hot Flashes." *Comprehensive Therapy* 31, no. 3 (2005): 224–36.

Pockaj, B. A., C. L. Loprinzi, J. A. Sloan, et al. "Pilot Evaluation of Black Cohosh for the Treatment of Hot Flashes in Women." *Cancer Investigation* 22, no. 4 (2004): 515–521.

Polyakov, N. G. *A Study of the Biological Activity of Infusions of Valerian and Motherwort and Their Mixtures.* Moscow: Information of the First All Russian Session of Pharmacists, 1964: 319–24.

Potts, B. *Witches Heal.* Ann Arbor, MI: DuReve, 1988.

Rahman, K., and G. M. Lowe. "Garlic and Cardiovascular Disease: A Critical Review." *Journal of Nutrition* 136, Suppl 3 (2006): 736S–40S.

Ringdahl, E., S. Pereira, J. Delzell. "Treatment of Primary Insomnia." *Journal of the American Board of Family Practice* 17 (2004): 212–19.

Ritz, S. "Growing Through Menopause." *Medical Self-Care* (Winter 1981): 70–74.

Rosen, R. C., and J. L. Barsky. "Normal Sexual Response in Women." *Obstetrics and Gynecology Clinics of North America* 33 (2006): 4515–26.

Rothenberg, R. *Medical Dictionary and Health Manual.* New York: Signet, 1983.

Samuels, M., and N. Samuels. *The Well Adult.* New York: Simon & Schuster, 1991.

Setchell, K., and E. Lydeking-Olsen. "Dietary Phytoestrogens and Their Effect on Bone: Evidence from in Vitro and in Vivo, Human Observational, and Dietary Intervention Studies." *American Journal of Clinical Nutrition* 78, Suppl (2003): 593S–609S.

Shabsigh, R., A. Anastasiades, K. L. Cooper, M. P. Rutman. "Female Sexual Dysfunction, Voiding Symptoms and Depression: Common Findings in Partners of Men with Erectile Dysfunction." *World Journal of Urology* 24 (2006): 6653–56.

Sharaf, A., et al. "Glycyrrhetic Acid as an Active Estrogenic Substance Separated from *Glycyrrhiza glabra* (liquorice)." *Egyptian Journal of Pharmaceutical Science 16*, no. 2 (1975): 245–51.

Shauenberg, P., and F. Paris. *Guide to Medicinal Plants.* New Canaan, CT: Keats, 1977.

Sloane, E. *Biology of Women,* 2d ed. Albany, NY: Delmar, 1985.

Smith, S. *"Vitex agnus-castus."* Pamphlet translated by the author, orig. in *Zeitschrift für Phytotherapie* (July 1986).

Speroff, L. "Efficacy and Tolerability of a Novel Estradiol Vaginal Ring for Relief of Menopausal Symptoms." *Obstetrics and Gynecology* 102, no. 4 (2003): 823–34.

Steinem, G. *Revolution from Within.* Boston: Little Brown, 1993.

Tang, B. M. P., G. D. Eslick, C. Nowson, C. Smith, A. Bensoussan. "Use of Calcium or Calcium in Combination with Vitamin D Supplementation to Prevent Fractures and Bone Loss in People Aged 50 Years and Older: A Meta-Analysis." *Lancet* 370, no. 9588 (2007): 657–66.

Tharakan, B., and B. Manyam. "Botanical Therapies in Sexual Dysfunction." *Phytotherapy Research* 19 (2005): 457–63.

Thurston, R. C., H. Joffe, C. N. Soares, B. L. Harlow. "Physical Activity and Risk of Vasomotor Symptoms in Women with and without a History of Depression: Results from the Harvard Study of Moods and Cycles." *Menopause* 13, no. 4 (2006): 553–60.

Tierra, L. *The Herbs of Life.* Freedom, CA: The Crossing Press, 1992.

Tierra, M., ed. *Essays on Herbalism; The American Herbalists Guild.* Freedom, CA: The Crossing Press, 1992.

———, ed. *Planetary Herbology.* Santa Fe: Lotus Press, 1988.

Vander, A. J., and D. S. Luciano. *Human Physiology,* 5th ed. New York: McGraw-Hill, 1980.

Verit, F. F., A. Verit, E. Yeni. "The Prevalence of Sexual Dysfunction and Associated Risk Factors in Women with Chronic Pelvic Pain: A Cross-Sectional Study." *Archives of Gynecology and Obstetrics* 274 (2006): 5297–302.

Viereck, V., G. Emons, W. Wuttke. "Black Cohosh: Just Another phytoestrogen?" *Trends in Endocrinology and Metabolism* 16, no. 5 (2005): 214–21.

Vogel, V. *American Indian Medicine.* Norman: University of Oklahoma Press, 1970.

Weed, S. *Wise Woman Ways: Menopausal Years.* Woodstock, NY: Ash Tree, 1992.

Weiss, R. F. *Herbal Medicine.* Beaconsfield, England: Beaconsfield, 1988.

Willett, W. *Eat, Drink, and Be Healthy.* Cambridge: Harvard University Press, 2002.

Williams, S. R. *Essentials of Nutrition and Diet Therapy,* 5th ed. New York: Times Mirror/Mosby, 1990.

Wood, M. *The Magical Staff.* Berkeley, CA: North Atlantic Books, 1992.

Wren, R. C. *Potter's New Cyclopedia,* 15th ed. Saffron Walden, UK: C. W. Daniel, 1988.

Zautra, A. J., and B. W. Smith. "Depression and Reactivity to Stress in Older Women with Rheumatoid Arthritis and Osteoarthritis." *Psychosomatic Medicine* 63 (2001): 687–96.

Index

digestive difficulties, 122–23
immune strength, 140–48
nervous system changes, 133–40
nutritional needs, 122–25
vaginal changes, 148–52
weight gain, 37, 114–15, 126
Potassium, 48–49, 51, 53
Pregnancy, 16–17, 76
Premarin, 95, 103
Premature ovarian failure, 9, 104
Prickly ash bark (Salix alba), 119
Progesterone
chaste berry and, 101
erratic menstrual cycles and, 16
herbal medicine for, 78, 98
for menopausal symptoms, 42
"natural," 102–3
role in reproductive process, 8–9
synthetic, 96
wild yam and, 99
Progestin, 95, 96
Protein, 14, 38, 49, 50, 132

R

Raspberry leaf (Rubus idaeus)
for heavy bleeding, 21
for improved intimacy, 151
for improving fertility, 23, 24
for moistening tissues, 80
for nervous system support, 58
Red clover flower (Trifolium pratense)
for coming off HRT, 107, 108
for improving fertility, 24
for moistening tissues, 80
phytoestrogens in, 100
Reproductive system pain. See also Migraines, menstrual
additional treatments, 67
Aromatherapy blend for pain, 67
chronic pelvic pain (CCP), 60–61
dysmenorrhea, 60, 62, 63
herbal medicine for, 61–63, 64
during intercourse, 62
nutrition for, 66
pelvic organ prolapse, 60, 149
severe, physical or emotional, 65–66
Resources, 175–80
Resveratrol, 38, 117, 148
Rheumatoid arthritis (RA), 114, 116–17

Roberts, Susan, 127
Rosehips (Rosa canina), 21, 24
Rosemary (Rosmarinus officinalis)
for cerebral circulation, 64
for colds and flu, 141
for dry hair, 89
for erratic cycles, 18
essential oil, 91
for headaches, 67
illustration, 171
for memory and mental clarity, 138, 139, 140
for skin changes, 88
Rose petals (Rosa species), 21, 28, 58
Rossouw, Jacques, 132–33

S

Sage leaf (Salvia officinalis)
for cerebral circulation, 64
for colds and flu, 141
for emotional lows, 59
for heavy bleeding, 21, 77
for keeping cool, 70
for pelvic pain, 61
toning vaginal tissues, 62
Salt, excess, 44, 50
Salves, herbal, 32, 84, 155
SAM-e (S-adenosylmethionine), 120
Samia and Fatima's Diamanda Special, 89–90
Sandalwood essential oil, 91
Sarsaparilla root (Smilax ornata), 24, 73, 79, 110
Senna, 62, 124
Serotonin, 116, 127
Sexual activity
benefits of, 78, 83
libido, 27–28, 78
pain during, 62
in perimenopause, 27–30
in postmenopause, 78, 148–49
Shatavari (Asparagus racemosa), 27, 28, 135, 150
Shepherd's purse (Capsella bursa-pastoris), 76
Shiitake mushrooms, 142, 148
Shingles, 145–48
Siberian ginseng, 135
Skin and hair
additional treatments, 92
aromatic skin and hair rinse, 91
dry hair conditioning formula, 89–90
herbal medicine for, 87, 88–91

U

Ulcerative colitis, 116, 117
Urinary-tract infection (UTI), 60, 81, 143–44
Uterine cancer, 96, 97, 98

V

Vaginal health
    additional treatments, 151–52
    douching, 29–30, 78–79, 84, 85
    herbal medicine for, 150–51
    infections, 29, 80–81, 84, 85, 149
    lubrication, 83, 149
    nutrition for, 83, 151
    perimenopausal, 27–30
    postmenopausal, 148–52
    tea for, 149–50
Vaginal thinning and drying
    about, 78–79, 149
    additional treatments, 83–85
    herbal medicine for, 62, 79–82
    natural approach, 103
    nutrition for, 83
Valerian root *(Valeriana officinalis)*
    illustration, 172
    for pelvic pain, 61
    reactions to, 61
    for reproductive pain, 63
    as sleep aid, 63, 66, 136–37, 138
Vasodilators, 68
Vegetarian diet, 25, 132
Vervain *(Verbena officinalis)*, 57, 173
Vibrel sex enhancement gel, 152
Violet flower *(Viola tricolor)*, 58
Visualization. *See also* Meditation
    for colds and flu, 143
    for improving fertility, 26
    for joint mobility, 123
    Ten-Minute Visualization, 20
Vitamin A, 148
Vitamin B$_6$, 39
Vitamin C, 14, 71, 72, 142, 148
Vitamin D, 25, 48, 49–50, 53
Vitamin E, 29, 43, 72, 83
Vitamin K, 48, 53
Vitamins, overusing, 39

W

Watercress, illustration, 173

Water retention and bloating, 39
Weight
    herbal medicine for, 128–30
    ideal, 126
    during menopause, 37
    nutrition for healthy weight, 131–32
    postmenopausal gain, 114–15, 126–27
Weight-bearing exercise, 47, 51
Weight loss
    for bone health, 54
    diet products, 127
    glycemic index (GI) and, 127
    herbs for, 129
    through fitness, 129
    tips for, 126
Wild oat *(Avena sativa)*, 52
Wild yam root *(Dioscorea villosa)*
    for depression, 56
    essential oil of, 30, 83
    herbal hormone in, 100
    herbal salve, vaginal, 32
    HRT and, 98–99
    for moistening tissues, 79
    "natural" progesterone and, 102–3
    for skin changes, 88
Willow bark *(Salix alba)*, 117, 118, 119
Wintergreen essential oil, 122
Women's Health Initiative, 115, 132

Y

Yarrow *(Achillea millefolium)*
    illustration, 174
    for joint health, 119
    for keeping cool, 70
    for night sweats and palpitations, 69
    toning vaginal tissues, 62
    for vaginal infections, 85
Yeast infections, 29, 84
Yellow dock root *(Rumex crispus)*, 52
Yellow mustard powder, 121–22
Yerba mansa root *(Anemopsis californica)*, 84
Yerba mate *(Ilex paraguaensis)*, 128, 129
Yoga, 25, 115

Z

Zestra, 152
Zinc, 83, 148

Printed in the United States
by Baker & Taylor Publisher Services